High Blood Pressure

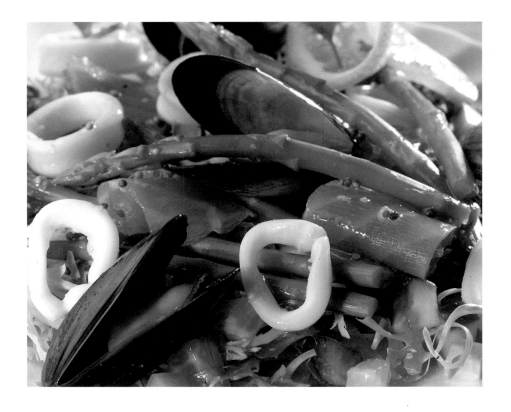

Recipes and Practical Advice for your Health

General Editor: Gina Steer

FLAME TREE
PUBLISHING

D0317184

Publisher & Creative Director: Nick Wells
Project Editor: Sarah Goulding
Designer: Mike Spender
With thanks to: Gina Steer

This is a **FLAME TREE** Book

FLAME TREE PUBLISHING
Crabtree Hall, Crabtree Lane
Fulham, London SW6 6TY
United Kingdom
www.flametreepublishing.com

Flame Tree is part of The Foundry Creative Media Company Limited

First published 2005

05 07 09 08 06
1 3 5 7 9 10 8 6 4 2

ISBN 1 84451 116 2

A copy of the CIP data for this book is available from the British Library.

Printed in Malaysia

Contents

Combatting High Blood Pressure   4–5

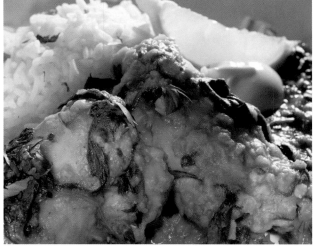

Aromatic Chicken Curry   6

Bean & Cashew Stir Fry   7

Bulghur Wheat Salad with Minty Lemon Dressing   8

Carrot, Celeriac & Sesame Seed Salad   9

Chicken Noodle Soup   10

Chinese Salad with Soy & Ginger Dressing   11

Chunky Halibut Casserole   12

Citrus Monkfish Kebabs   13

Citrus-grilled Plaice   14

Cod with Fennel & Cardamom   15

Cream of Spinach Soup   16

Curly Endive & Seafood Salad   17

Fish Roulades with Rice & Spinach   18

Gingered Cod Steaks   19

Griddled Garlic & Lemon Squid   20

Haddock with an Olive Crust   21

Hot Salsa-filled Sole   22

Jamaican Jerk Pork with Rice & Peas   23

Marinated Vegetable Kebabs   24

Mediterranean Potato Salad   25

Mexican Chicken   26

Mixed Vegetables Stir Fry   27

Pad Thai   28

Paella   29

Pasta with Courgettes, Rosemary & Lemon   30

Peperonata   31

Pumpkin & Chickpea Curry   32

Ratatouille Mackerel   33

Rice with Smoked Salmon & Ginger   34

Rice with Squash & Sage   35

Rich Tomato Soup with Roasted Red Peppers   36

Salmon Noisettes with Fruity Sauce   37

Salmon with Herbed Potatoes   38

Sardines with Redcurrants   39

Spiced Couscous & Vegetables   40

Spicy Cucumber Stir Fry   41

Steamed Whole Trout with Ginger & Spring Onion   42

Stir-fried Chicken with Spinach, Tomatoes & Pine Nuts   43

Thai Noodles & Vegetables with Tofu   44

Thai Stir-fried Noodles   45

Turkey & Tomato Tagine   46

Turkey with Oriental Mushrooms   47

Zesty Whole-baked Fish   48

Combatting High Blood Pressure

With our changing eating habits and lifestyle, high blood pressure is becoming more and more prevalent in the West. Medical experts attribute this in many cases to bad diet. In recent years we have been eating an increasing amount of processed convenience foods, relying on the freezer and microwave for our meals and eating take-away foods from fish and chips, burgers, and kebabs to pizza, Indian and Chinese food. This is coupled with an increase in sugary fizzy drinks, alcohol drinking, sweets, biscuits, cakes, crisps and instant snacks, designed to satisfy hunger pangs in a flash with no regard to the nutritional cost. Together with the majority of people not taking enough exercise – relying on the car rather than walking, sitting in front of the television or computer rather than playing sport – is it any wonder that for many our hearts are having a serious problem coping? The remedy is simple – we need to cut out the junk food, return to a well-cooked, nutritionally balanced diet and take regular exercise.

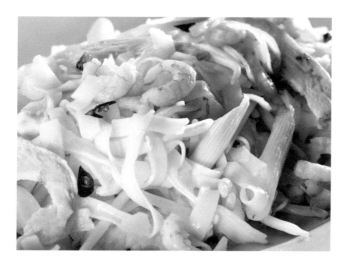

Our bodies rely totally on our hearts. It is the largest muscle in our body and controls the flow of blood. The heart pumps the five litres of blood that our body contains through the arteries into tiny capillaries which feed the body tissues before returning to the heart back through the veins (the circulatory system). This happens 75 times every single minute. An accurate indication of how healthy your heart is can be assessed by taking your blood pressure, essentially a measurement of how your heart is performing. There are two readings taken: the higher measurement records the blood flow at its peak while the heart is beating, and the lower measurement records the flow of blood when the heart is relaxing. An average normal reading is 120/80, but obviously there are always variations on this measurement.

As we grow older, the elasticity in the veins and arteries can reduce. Healthy veins and arteries expand and contract easily and the blood flows freely, but when, either due to poor health or age, they no longer work efficiently, high blood pressure occurs. Eating badly can thicken the arteries and have the same effect, making it harder for blood to get round the body, raising the pressure in the arteries and increasing the risk of problems. This can also happen on a temporary basis when you get upset, excited or frightened. The heart beats faster, pushing the blood more quickly round the body, and if the elasticity has decreased then a problem can occur such as stroke, heart attack or blood clots. However, there are steps that can be taken to either prevent or reduce this lack of elasticity, and that is by watching the diet.

As with all diseases, a healthy lifestyle is paramount to a healthy life and ensuring the body's organs work efficiently. If you have been diagnosed with high blood pressure, or your family have a history of heart problems, then it is essential that you look at your lifestyle and change it if necessary.

Many health experts believe that we eat too much salt, and this is a contributory factor in high blood pressure. The average body will get sufficient salt from a balanced diet but in the West on average we consume an extra 10–12 grams each day. Simply by reducing this amount, we are well on the way to addressing the problem. Try not putting salt in your food when it is being cooked, and instead use herbs or spices to flavour. You will be surprised how quickly your palate adjusts.

Preparing and cooking healthy dishes need not be a chore, and there are plenty of recipes that can be on the table in less than 30 minutes and will be tasty, more nutritious and satisfying than any take-away or fast food. You will also have the satisfaction of knowing that these dishes are doing you and your family's hearts good by either preventing or reducing high blood pressure.

To further reduce the risk of high blood pressure, there are a few simple rules to observe. Firstly it is vital to reduce the intake of all saturated fat, butter, lard, dripping, cream, whole milk, hard cheese and the fat from meats. Buy only lean meats and remove any fat before cooking. Remove the skin from poultry, as any fat in poultry is situated immediately under the skin. Use monounsaturated oils for cooking such as olive, soya or sunflower oil, but use sparingly and ban fried foods – especially deep fried foods – for ever.

Include plenty of oily fish in your diet, such as mackerel, kippers, pilchards, sardines, salmon and trout. They are high in omega-3 fatty acids, an unsaturated fat that will help to eliminate the bad LDL cholesterol in your blood. It has been suggested that 115 g of oily fish 2–3 times a week dramatically reduces heart problems.

Most of us love pastries, cakes and biscuits, but unfortunately these are bad for us and need to be drastically cut back or eliminated. Limit the amount of sugary foods you eat – try keeping a slice of cake or a biscuit as a treat rather than the norm, and that way it will be more enjoyable and is one more step to a healthy lifestyle. It is not all bad news, though – there are plenty of delicious foods that can be eaten and will help maintain a healthy heart.

Increase your intake of high fibre foods, as these are not only extremely good for the body but they also help to keep the stomach feeling full and satiated, reducing the need for snacking on sugary sweets or salty snacks.

Vegetables, fruit, pulses, rice and wholegrain cereals should all be eaten regularly. Soya beans and soya oil have proven to be very beneficial for the heart, and here in the West we tend to discount this very important food. Soya milk is also nutritionally excellent and if switched with whole milk would make a substantial difference to blood pressure levels.

For many there is a real bonus – it has been found that beer and wine drunk in moderation (and that is the key word – moderation!) – can play an important part in the diet. One glass of red wine or beer can help the cholesterol levels within the blood, thus improving blood pressure. Any benefits of this are negated by drinking to excess, though, so try not to over-indulge.

Lifestyle choices can also help to reduce high blood pressure. Try and spend more time relaxing and avoid stress wherever possible. Exercise more, starting slowly and gradually increasing how much you do. It is recommended that the heart needs to work faster for at least 20–30 minutes, three or four times a week but ideally each day for there to be an improvement. If you don't enjoy or are not capable of intensive exercise, a brisk walk every day will be just as beneficial. Finally, giving up smoking should be of paramount importance in your quest for a healthy heart.

To help your healthy lifestyle, this book provides lots of delicious recipes that are easy to prepare and cook and ensure that flavour is not sacrificed for health. With tasty dishes from Aromatic Chicken Curry to Citrus Monkfish Kebabs and Paella, you'll soon be on your way to a healthy heart.

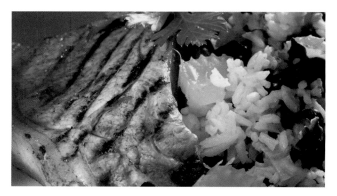

Aromatic Chicken Curry

Nutritional details

per 100 g

energy	138 kcals/580 kj
protein	12 g
carbohydrate	13 g
fat	4 g
fibre	0.6 g
sugar	0.2 g
sodium	0.2 g

Ingredients   Serves 4

125 g/4 oz red lentils
2 tsp ground coriander
½ tsp cumin seeds
2 tsp mild curry paste
1 bay leaf
small strip of lemon rind
600 ml/1 pint chicken
    or vegetable stock
8 chicken thighs, skinned
175 g/6 oz spinach leaves,
    rinsed and shredded
1 tbsp freshly
    chopped coriander
2 tsp lemon juice
freshly ground
    black pepper

To serve:
freshly cooked rice
low fat natural yogurt

Step-by-step guide

1 Put the lentils in a sieve and rinse thoroughly under cold running water.

2 Dry-fry the ground coriander and cumin seeds in a large saucepan over a low heat for about 30 seconds. Stir in the curry paste.

3 Add the lentils to the saucepan with the bay leaf and lemon rind, then pour in the stock.

4 Stir, then slowly bring to the boil. Turn down the heat, half cover the pan with a lid and simmer gently for 5 minutes, stirring occasionally.

5 Secure the chicken thighs with cocktail sticks to keep their shape. Place in the pan and half cover. Simmer for 15 minutes.

6 Stir in the shredded spinach and cook for a further 25 minutes or until the chicken is very tender and the sauce is thick.

7 Remove the bay leaf and lemon rind. Stir in the coriander and lemon juice, then season to taste with pepper. Serve immediately with the rice and a little natural yogurt.

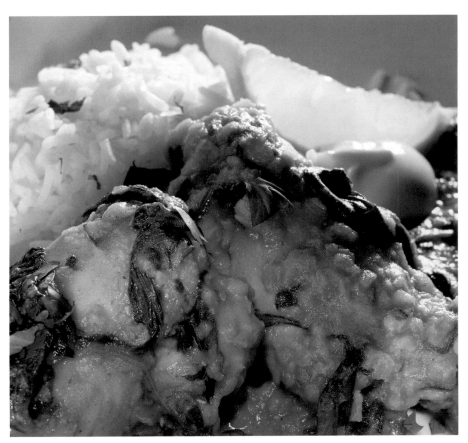

✓ cows' milk-free   ✓ egg-free   ✓ gluten-free   ✓ wheat-free   ✓ nut-free   ✓ vegetarian   ✓ vegan   ✓ seafood-free

Bean & Cashew Stir Fry

Nutritional details

per 100 g

energy	129 kcals/537 kj
protein	3 g
carbohydrate	9 g
fat	10 g
fibre	1.9 g
sugar	3.1 g
sodium	0.3 g

Ingredients   Serves 4

3 tbsp sunflower oil
1 onion, peeled and finely chopped
1 celery stalk, trimmed
    and chopped
2.5 cm/1 inch piece fresh root
    ginger, peeled and grated
2 garlic cloves, peeled and crushed
1 red chilli, deseeded and
    finely chopped
175 g/6 oz fine French beans,
    trimmed and halved
175 g/6 oz mangetout,
    sliced diagonally into 3
75 g/3 oz unsalted cashew nuts
1 tsp brown sugar
125 ml/4 fl oz vegetable stock
2 tbsp dry sherry
1 tbsp light soy sauce
1 tsp red wine vinegar
freshly ground
    black pepper
freshly chopped coriander,
    to garnish

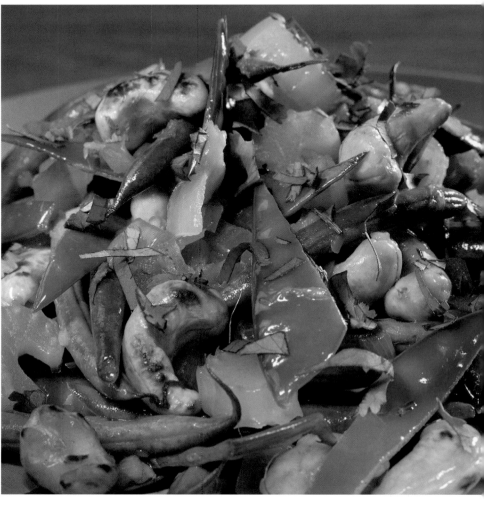

Step-by-step guide

1   Heat a wok or large frying pan, add the oil and when hot, add the onion and celery and stir-fry gently for 3–4 minutes or until softened.

2   Add the ginger, garlic and chilli to the wok and stir-fry for 30 seconds. Stir in the French beans and mangetout together with the cashew nuts and continue to stir-fry for 1–2 minutes, or until the nuts are golden brown.

3   Dissolve the sugar in the stock, then blend with the sherry, soy sauce and vinegar. Stir into the bean mixture and bring to the boil. Simmer gently, stirring occasionally for 3–4 minutes, or until the beans and mangetout are tender but still crisp and the sauce has thickened slightly. Season to taste with pepper. Transfer to a warmed serving bowl or spoon on to individual plates. Sprinkle with freshly chopped coriander and serve immediately.

✓ cows' milk-free   ✓ egg-free   ✓ gluten-free   ✓ wheat-free   ✓ nut-free   ✓ vegetarian   ✓ vegan   ✓ seafood-free

Bulghur Wheat Salad with Minty Lemon Dressing

Nutritional details

per 100 g

energy	65 kcals/270 kj
protein	2 g
carbohydrate	8 g
fat	3 g
fibre	0.8 g
sugar	3.4 g
sodium	0.3 g

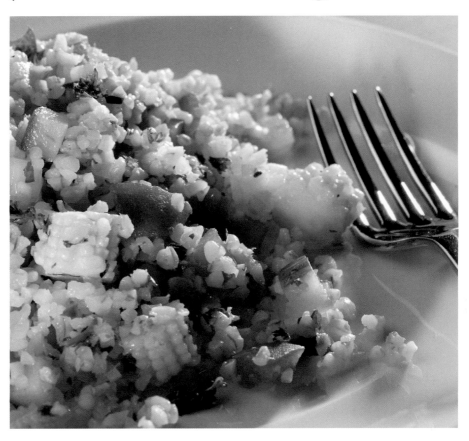

Ingredients   Serves 4

125 g/4 oz bulghur wheat
10 cm /4 inch piece cucumber
2 shallots, peeled
125 g/4 oz baby sweetcorn
3 ripe but firm tomatoes

For the dressing:
grated rind of 1 lemon
3 tbsp lemon juice
3 tbsp freshly
   chopped mint
2 tbsp freshly
   chopped parsley
1–2 tsp clear honey
2 tbsp sunflower oil
freshly ground
   black pepper

Step-by-step guide

1 Place the bulghur wheat in a saucepan and cover with boiling water.

2 Simmer for about 10 minutes, then drain thoroughly and turn into a serving bowl.

3 Cut the cucumber into small cubes, chop the shallots finely and reserve. Steam the sweetcorn over a pan of boiling water for 10 minutes or until tender. Drain and slice into thick chunks.

4 Cut a cross on the top of each tomato and place in boiling water until their skins start to peel away.

5 Remove the skins and the seeds and cut the tomatoes into small cubes.

6 Make the dressing by briskly whisking all the ingredients in a small bowl until mixed well.

7 When the bulghur wheat has cooled a little, add all the prepared vegetables and stir in the dressing. Season to taste with pepper and serve.

cows' milk-free   egg-free   gluten-free   wheat-free   nut-free   vegetarian   vegan   seafood-free

Carrot, Celeriac & Sesame Seed Salad

Nutritional details

per 100 g

energy	95 kcals/395 kj
protein	1 g
carbohydrate	18 g
fat	3 g
fibre	trace
sugar	5.1 g
sodium	trace

Ingredients   Serves 6

225 g/8 oz celeriac
225 g/8 oz carrots, peeled
50 g/2 oz seedless raisins
2 tbsp sesame seeds
freshly chopped parsley, to garnish

For the lemon & chilli dressing:
grated rind of 1 lemon
4 tbsp lemon juice
2 tbsp sunflower oil
2 tbsp clear honey
1 red bird's eye chilli, deseeded
    and finely chopped
freshly ground black pepper

Step-by-step guide

1 Slice the celeriac into thin matchsticks. Place in a small saucepan of boiling salted water and boil for 2 minutes.

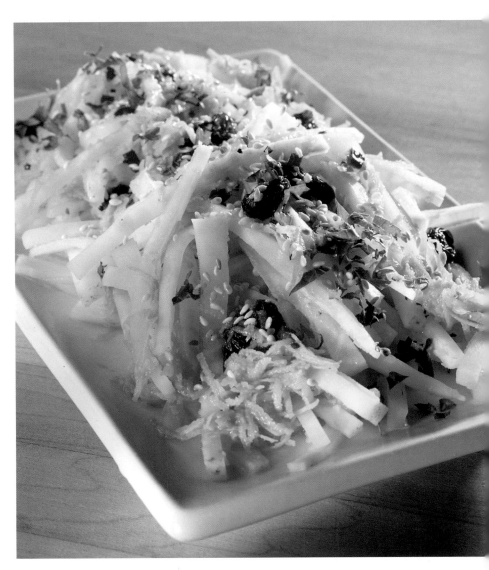

2 Drain and rinse the celeriac in cold water and place in a mixing bowl.

3 Finely grate the carrot. Add the carrot and the raisins to the celeriac in the bowl.

4 Place the sesame seeds under a hot grill or dry-fry in a frying pan for 1–2 minutes until golden brown, then leave to cool.

5 Make the dressing by whisking together the lemon rind, lemon juice, oil, honey, chilli and seasoning or by shaking thoroughly in a screw-topped jar.

6 Pour 2 tablespoons of the dressing over the salad and toss well. Turn into a serving dish and sprinkle over the toasted sesame seeds and chopped parsley. Serve the remaining dressing separately.

Chicken Noodle Soup

Nutritional details

per 100 g

energy	43 kcals/182 kj
protein	5 g
carbohydrate	4 g
fat	0.8 g
fibre	0.9 g
sugar	2.1 g
sodium	trace

   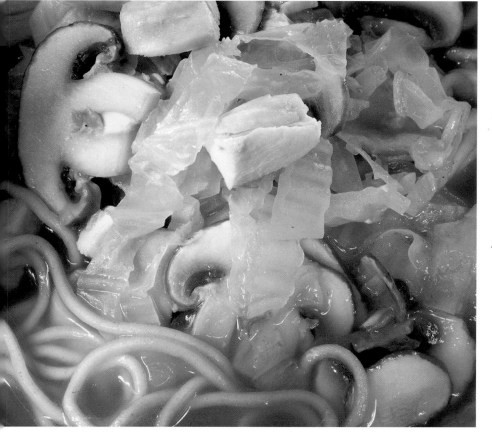

Ingredients   Serves 4

carcass of a medium-sized
  cooked chicken
1 large carrot, peeled and
  roughly chopped
1 medium onion, peeled
  and quartered
1 leek, trimmed and roughly chopped
2–3 bay leaves
a few black peppercorns
2 litres/3½ pints water
225 g/8 oz Chinese cabbage,
  trimmed
50 g/2 oz chestnut mushrooms,
  wiped and sliced
125 g/4 oz cooked chicken,
  sliced or chopped
50 g/2 oz medium or fine egg
  thread noodles

Step-by-step guide

1 Break the chicken carcass into smaller pieces and place in a wok with the carrot, onion, leek, bay leaves, peppercorns and water. Bring slowly to the boil. Skim away any fat or scum that rises for the first 15 minutes. Simmer very gently for 1–1½ hours. If the liquid reduces by more than one third, add a little more water.

2 Remove from the heat and leave until cold. Strain into a large bowl and chill in the refrigerator until any fat in the stock rises and sets on the surface. Remove the fat and discard. Draw a sheet of absorbent kitchen paper across the surface of the stock to absorb any remaining fat.

3 Return the stock to the wok and bring to a simmer. Add the Chinese cabbage, mushrooms and chicken and simmer gently for 7–8 minutes until the vegetables are tender.

4 Meanwhile, cook the noodles according to the packet directions until tender. Drain well. Transfer a portion of noodles to each serving bowl before pouring in some soup and vegetables. Serve immediately.

✓ cows' milk-free   ✓ egg-free   ✓ gluten-free   ✓ wheat-free   ✓ nut-free   ✓ vegetarian   ✓ vegan   ✓ seafood-free

Chinese Salad with Soy & Ginger Dressing

Nutritional details

per 100 g

energy	73 kcals/306 kj
protein	2 g
carbohydrate	12 g
fat	2 g
fibre	0.6 g
sugar	1.2 g
sodium	0.5 g

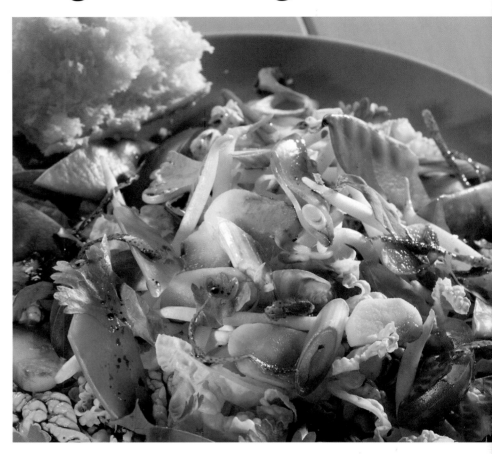

Ingredients   Serves 4

1 head of Chinese cabbage
200 g can water chestnuts,
    drained
6 spring onions, trimmed
4 ripe but firm cherry tomatoes
125 g/4 oz mangetout
125 g/4 oz beansprouts
2 tbsp freshly
    chopped coriander

For the soy and ginger dressing:
2 tbsp sunflower oil
2 tbsp light soy sauce
2.5 cm/1 inch piece root ginger,
    peeled and finely grated
zest and juice of 1 lemon
freshly ground black pepper
crusty white bread,
    to serve

Step-by-step guide

1 Rinse and finely shred the Chinese cabbage and place in a serving dish.

2 Slice the water chestnuts into small slivers and cut the spring onions diagonally into 2.5 cm/ 1 inch lengths, then split lengthwise into thin strips.

3 Cut the tomatoes in half and then slice each half into three wedges and reserve.

4 Simmer the mangetout in boiling water for 2 minutes until beginning to soften, drain and cut in half diagonally.

5 Arrange the water chestnuts, spring onions, mangetout, tomatoes and beansprouts on top of the shredded Chinese cabbage. Garnish with the freshly chopped coriander.

6 Make the dressing by whisking all the ingredients together in a small bowl until mixed thoroughly. Serve with the bread and the salad.

Chunky Halibut Casserole

Nutritional details

per 100 g

energy	72 kcals/307 kj
protein	6 g
carbohydrate	11 g
fat	1 g
fibre	0.9 g
sugar	2.1 g
sodium	trace

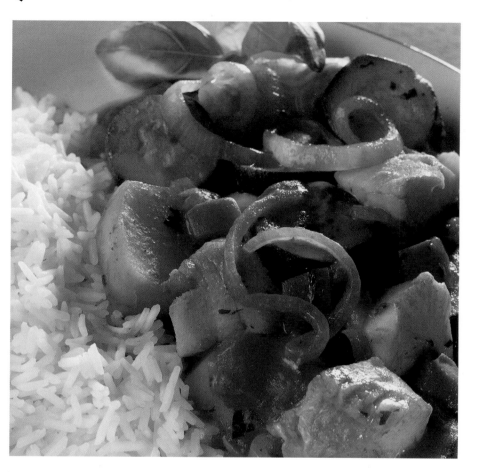

Ingredients   Serves 6

1 tbsp olive oil
2 large onions, peeled and
   sliced into rings
1 red pepper, deseeded and
   roughly chopped
450 g/1 lb potatoes, peeled
450 g/1 lb courgettes, trimmed
   and thickly sliced
2 tbsp plain flour
1 tbsp paprika
2 tsp vegetable oil
150 ml/¼ pint fish stock
400 g can chopped tomatoes
2 tbsp freshly chopped basil
freshly ground
   black pepper
450 g/1 lb halibut fillet,
   skinned and cut into
   2.5 cm/ 1 inch cubes
sprigs of fresh basil,
   to garnish
freshly cooked rice,
   to serve

Step-by-step guide

1 Heat the oil in a large saucepan, add the onions and pepper and cook for 5 minutes, or until softened.

2 Cut the peeled potatoes into 2.5 cm/1 inch cubes, rinse lightly and shake dry, then add them to the onions and pepper in the saucepan. Add the courgettes and cook, stirring frequently, for a further 2–3 minutes.

3 Sprinkle the flour, paprika and vegetable oil into the saucepan and cook, stirring continuously, for 1 minute. Pour in the stock and the chopped tomatoes, and bring to the boil.

4 Add the basil to the casserole, season to taste with pepper and cover. Simmer for 15 minutes, then add the halibut and simmer very gently for a further 5–7 minutes, or until the fish and vegetables are just tender.

5 Garnish with basil sprigs and serve immediately with freshly cooked rice.

✓ cows' milk-free   ✓ egg-free   ✓ gluten-free   ✓ wheat-free   ✓ nut-free   ✓ vegetarian   ✓ vegan   ✓ seafood-free

Citrus Monkfish Kebabs

Nutritional details

per 100 g

energy	95 kcals/396 kj
protein	15 g
carbohydrate	2 g
fat	3 g
fibre	0.2 g
sugar	0.3 g
sodium	0.2 g

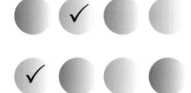

Ingredients   Serves 4

For the marinade:
1 tbsp sunflower oil
finely grated rind and
    juice of 1 lime
1 tbsp lemon juice
1 sprig of freshly
    chopped rosemary
1 tbsp wholegrain mustard
1 garlic clove, peeled
    and crushed
freshly ground
    black pepper

For the kebabs:
450 g/1 lb monkfish tail
8 raw tiger prawns
1 small green courgette,
    trimmed and sliced
4 tbsp of half-fat
    crème fraîche

Step-by-step guide

1   Preheat the grill and line the grill rack with tinfoil. Mix all the marinade ingredients together in a small bowl and reserve.

2   Using a sharp knife, cut down both sides of the monkfish tail. Remove the bone and discard. Cut away and discard any skin, then cut the monkfish into bite-sized cubes.

3   Peel the prawns, leaving the tails intact and remove the thin black vein that runs down the back of each prawn. Place the fish and prawns in a shallow dish.

4   Pour the marinade over the fish and prawns. Cover lightly and leave to marinate in the refrigerator for 30 minutes. Spoon the marinade over the fish and prawns occasionally during this time. Soak the skewers in cold water for 30 minutes, then drain.

5   Thread the cubes of fish, prawns and courgettes on to the drained skewers.

6   Arrange on the grill rack then place under the preheated grill and cook for 5–7 minutes, or until cooked thoroughly and the prawns have turned pink. Occasionally brush with the remaining marinade and turn the kebabs during cooking.

7   Mix 2 tablespoons of marinade with the crème fraîche and serve as a dip with the kebabs.

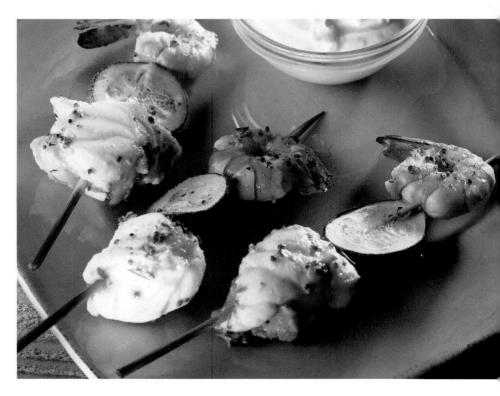

✓ cows' milk-free   ✓ egg-free   ✓ gluten-free   ✓ wheat-free   ✓ nut-free   ✓ vegetarian   ✓ vegan   ✓ seafood-free

Citrus-grilled Plaice

Nutritional details

per 100 g

energy	74 kcals/313 kj
protein	8 g
carbohydrate	8 g
fat	1 g
fibre	0.4 g
sugar	1.4 g
sodium	0.1 g

Ingredients   Serves 4

1 tsp sunflower oil
1 onion, peeled and chopped
1 orange pepper, deseeded
    and chopped
175 g/6 oz long-grain rice
150 ml/¼ pint orange juice
2 tbsp lemon juice
225 ml/8 fl oz vegetable stock
spray of oil
4 x 175 g/6 oz plaice fillets, skinned
1 orange
1 lemon
25 g/1 oz half-fat butter or
    low fat spread
2 tbsp freshly chopped tarragon
freshly ground
    black pepper
lemon wedges, to garnish

Step-by-step guide

1 Heat the oil in a large frying pan, then sauté the onion, pepper and rice for 2 minutes.

2 Add the orange and lemon juice and bring to the boil. Reduce the heat, add half the stock and simmer for 15–20 minutes, or until the rice is tender, adding the remaining stock as necessary.

3 Preheat the grill. Finely spray the base of the grill pan with oil. Place the plaice fillets in the base and reserve.

4 Finely grate the orange and lemon rind. Squeeze the juice from half of each fruit.

5 Melt the butter or low-fat spread in a small saucepan. Add the grated rind and juice and half of the tarragon and use to baste the plaice fillets.

6 Cook one side only of the fish under the preheated grill at a medium heat for 4–6 minutes, basting continuously.

7 Once the rice is cooked, stir in the remaining tarragon and season to taste with pepper. Garnish the fish with the lemon wedges and serve immediately with the rice.

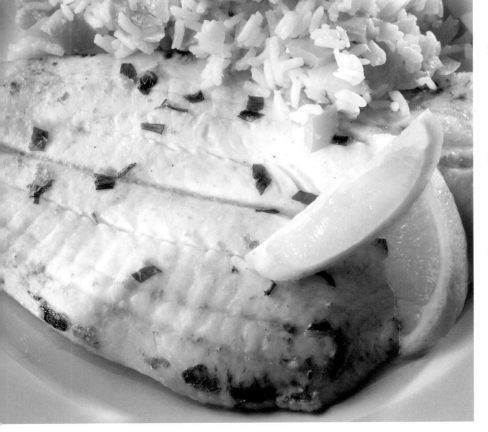

cows' milk-free   egg-free   gluten-free   wheat-free   nut-free   vegetarian   vegan   seafood-free

Cod with Fennel & Cardamom

Nutritional details

per 100 g

energy	89 kcals/378 kj
protein	16 g
carbohydrate	3 g
fat	2 g
fibre	trace
sugar	none
sodium	0.3 g

Ingredients   Serves 4

1 garlic clove, peeled
    and crushed
finely grated rind of 1 lemon
1 tsp lemon juice
1 tbsp olive oil
1 fennel bulb
1 tbsp cardamom pods
freshly ground
    black pepper
4 x 175 g/6 oz thick cod fillets

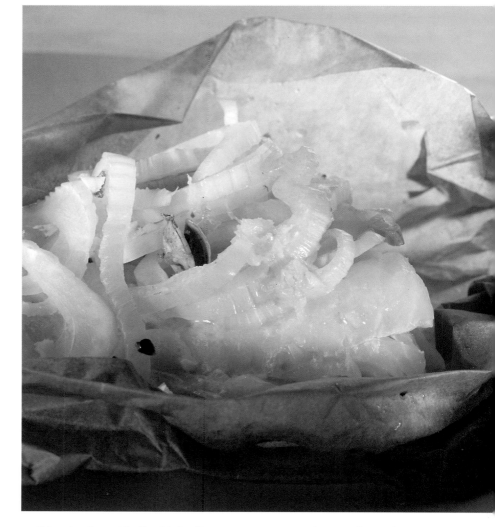

Step-by-step guide

1 Preheat the oven to 190°C/375°F/ Gas Mark 5. Place the garlic in a small bowl with the lemon rind and juice and the olive oil and stir well.

2 Cover and leave to infuse for at least 30 minutes. Stir well.

3 Trim the fennel bulb, thinly slice and place in a bowl.

4 Place the cardamom pods in a pestle and mortar and lightly pound to crack the pods.

5 Alternatively place in a polythene bag and pound gently with a rolling pin. Add the crushed cardamom to the fennel slices.

6 Season the fish with pepper and place on to four separate 20.5 x

20.5 cm/8 x 8 inch parchment paper squares.

7 Spoon the fennel mixture over the fish and drizzle with the infused oil.

8 Place the parcels on a baking sheet and bake in the preheated oven for 8–10 minutes or until cooked. Serve immediately in the paper parcels.

cows' milk-free   egg-free   gluten-free   wheat-free   nut-free   vegetarian   vegan   seafood-free

Cream of Spinach Soup

Nutritional details

per 100 g

energy	45 kcals/192 kj
protein	3 g
carbohydrate	8 g
fat	0.6 g
fibre	1 g
sugar	3.2 g
sodium	trace

Ingredients   Serves 6–8

1 large onion, peeled
    and chopped
5 large plump garlic cloves,
    peeled and chopped
2 medium potatoes,
    peeled and chopped
750 ml/1¼ pints cold water
450 g/1 lb spinach, washed
    and large stems removed
50 g/2 oz low fat butter
3 tbsp flour
750 ml/1¼ pints skimmed milk
½ tsp freshly grated nutmeg
freshly ground black pepper
6–8 tbsp half fat crème fraîche or
    soured cream
warm foccacia bread,
    to serve

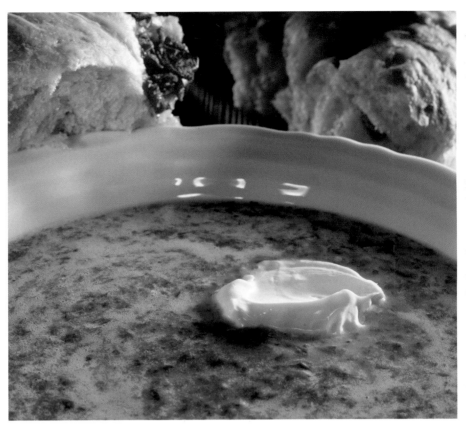

Step-by-step guide

1 Place the onion, garlic and potatoes in a large saucepan and cover with the cold water. Bring to the boil, then cover and simmer for 15–20 minutes, or until the potatoes are tender. Remove from the heat and add the spinach. Cover and set aside for 10 minutes.

2 Slowly melt the butter in another saucepan, add the flour and cook over a low heat for about 2 minutes. Remove the saucepan from the heat and add the milk, a little at a time, stirring continuously. Return to the heat and cook, stirring continuously, for 5–8 minutes, or until the sauce is smooth and slightly thickened. Add the freshly grated nutmeg, or to taste.

3 Blend the cooled potato and spinach mixture in a food processor or blender to a smooth purée, then return to the saucepan and gradually stir in the white sauce. Season to taste with pepper and gently reheat, taking care not to allow the soup to boil. Ladle into soup bowls and top with spoonfuls of crème fraîche or soured cream. Serve immediately with warm foccacia bread.

✓ cows' milk-free   ✓ egg-free   ✓ gluten-free   ✓ wheat-free   ✓ nut-free   ✓ vegetarian   ✓ vegan   ✓ seafood-free

Curly Endive & Seafood Salad

Nutritional details

per 100 g

energy	71 kcals/296 kj
protein	8 g
carbohydrate	4 g
fat	3 g
fibre	trace
sugar	0.4 g
sodium	0.3 g

Ingredients   Serves 4

1 head of curly endive lettuce
2 green peppers
12.5 cm/5 inch piece cucumber
125 g/4 oz squid, cleaned and
    cut into thin rings
225 g/8 oz baby asparagus spears
125 g/4 oz smoked salmon slices,
    cut into wide strips
175 g/6 oz fresh cooked mussels
    in their shells

For the lemon dressing:

2 tbsp sunflower oil
1 tbsp white wine vinegar
5 tbsp fresh lemon juice
1–2 tsp caster sugar
1 tsp mild whole-grain mustard
freshly ground
    black pepper

To garnish:

slices of lemon
sprigs of fresh coriander

Step-by-step guide

1   Rinse and tear the endive into small pieces and arrange on a serving platter.

2   Remove the seeds from the peppers and cut the peppers and the cucumber into small cubes. Sprinkle over the endive.

3   Bring a saucepan of water to the boil and add the squid rings. Bring the pan up to the boil again, then switch off the heat and leave it to stand for 5 minutes. Then drain and rinse thoroughly in cold water.

4   Cook the asparagus in boiling water for 5 minutes or until tender but just crisp. Arrange with the squid, smoked salmon and mussels on top of the salad.

5   To make the lemon dressing, put all the ingredients into a screw-topped jar or into a small bowl and mix thoroughly until the ingredients are combined.

6   Spoon 3 tablespoons of the dressing over the salad and serve the remainder in a small jug. Garnish the salad with slices of lemon and sprigs of coriander and serve.

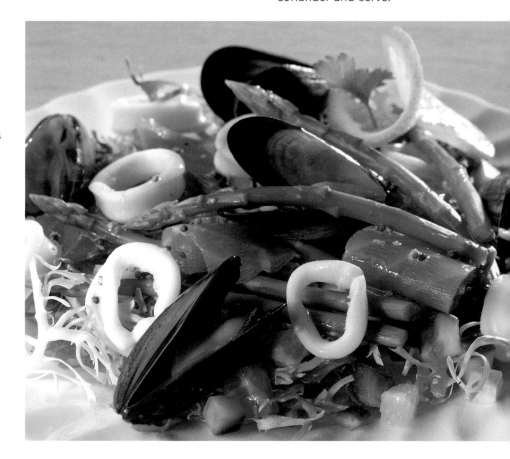

✓ cows' milk-free   ✓ egg-free   ✓ gluten-free   ✓ wheat-free   ✓ nut-free   ✓ vegetarian   ✓ vegan   ✓ seafood-free

Fish Roulades with Rice & Spinach

Nutritional details

per 100 g

energy	44 kcals/184 kj
protein	7 g
carbohydrate	2 g
fat	0.7 g
fibre	1.1 g
sugar	1 g
sodium	trace

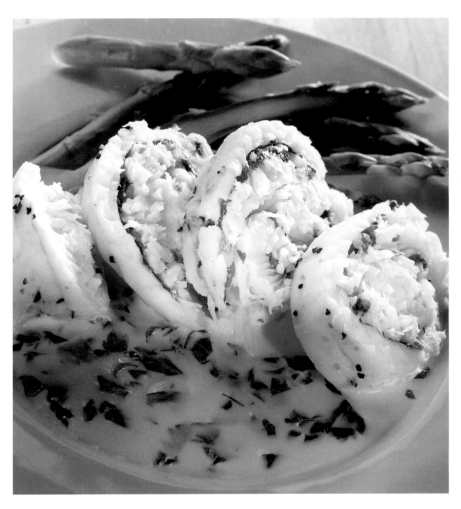

Ingredients   Serves 4

4 x 175 g/6 oz lemon sole, skinned
freshly ground black pepper
1 tsp fennel seeds
75 g/3 oz long-grain rice, cooked
150 g/5 oz white crab meat,
    fresh or canned
125 g/4 oz baby spinach,
    washed and trimmed
5 tbsp dry white wine
5 tbsp half-fat crème fraîche
2 tbsp freshly chopped parsley,
    plus extra to garnish
asparagus spears, to serve

Step-by-step guide

1   Wipe each fish fillet with either a clean damp cloth or kitchen paper. Place on a chopping board, skinned side up and season lightly with black pepper.

2   Place the fennel seeds in a pestle and mortar and crush lightly. Transfer to a small bowl and stir in the cooked rice. Drain the crab meat thoroughly. Add to the rice mixture and mix lightly.

3   Lay 2–3 spinach leaves over each fillet and top with a quarter of the crab meat mixture. Roll up and secure with a cocktail stick if necessary. Place into a large pan and pour over the wine. Cover and cook on a medium heat for 5–7 minutes or until cooked.

4   Remove the fish from the cooking liquid, and transfer to a serving plate and keep warm. Stir the crème fraîche into the cooking liquid and season to taste. Heat for 3 minutes, then stir in the chopped parsley.

5   Spoon the sauce on to the base of a plate. Cut each roulade into slices and arrange on top of the sauce. Serve with freshly cooked asparagus spears.

cows' milk-free   egg-free   gluten-free   wheat-free   nut-free   vegetarian   vegan   seafood-free

Gingered Cod Steaks

Nutritional details

per 100 g

energy	82 kcals/351 kj
protein	11 g
carbohydrate	8 g
fat	1.1 g
fibre	1 g
sugar	2.1 g
sodium	0.2 g

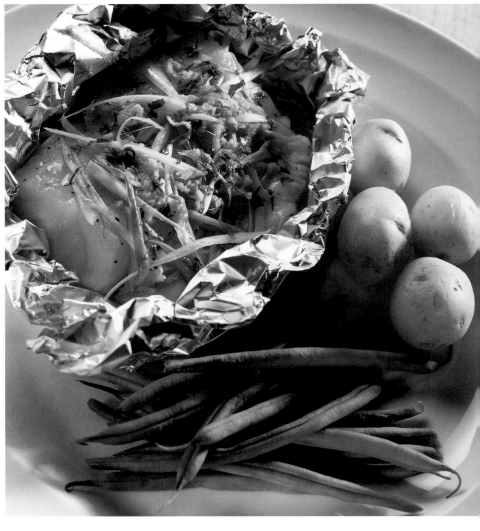

Ingredients   Serves 4

2.5 cm/1 inch piece
    fresh root ginger, peeled
4 spring onions
2 tsp freshly chopped parsley
1 tbsp soft brown sugar
4 x 175 g/6 oz thick
    cod steaks
freshly ground
    black pepper
3 tsp olive oil
freshly cooked vegetables,
    to serve

Step-by-step guide

1 Preheat the grill and line the grill rack with a layer of tinfoil. Coarsely grate the piece of ginger. Trim the spring onions and cut into thin strips.

2 Mix the spring onions, ginger, chopped parsley and sugar. Add 1 tablespoon of water.

3 Wipe the fish steaks. Season to taste with pepper. Place on to four separate 20.5 x 20.5 cm/8 x 8 inch tinfoil squares.

4 Carefully spoon the spring onions and ginger mixture over the fish. Drizzle the olive oil over the fish.

5 Loosely fold the foil over the steaks to enclose the fish and make a parcel.

6 Place under the preheated grill and cook for 10–12 minutes or until cooked and the flesh has turned opaque.

7 Place the fish parcels on individual serving plates. Serve immediately with the freshly cooked vegetables.

Griddled Garlic & Lemon Squid

Nutritional details

per 100 g

energy	96 kcals/403 kj
protein	10 g
carbohydrate	11 g
fat	1 g
fibre	0.1 g
sugar	0.2 g
sodium	0.2 g

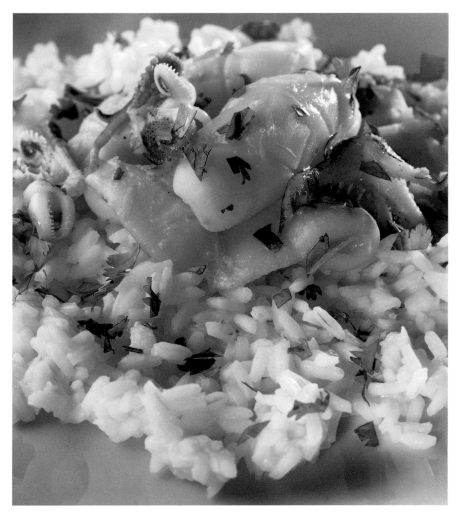

Ingredients Serves 4

125 g/4 oz long-grain rice
300 ml/½ pint fish stock
225 g/8 oz squid, cleaned
finely grated rind of 1 lemon
1 garlic clove, peeled
   and crushed
1 shallot, peeled and
   finely chopped
2 tbsp freshly chopped coriander
2 tbsp lemon juice
freshly ground
   black pepper

Step-by-step guide

1 Rinse the rice until the water runs clear, then place in a saucepan with the stock.

2 Bring to the boil, then reduce the heat. Cover and simmer gently for 10 minutes.

3 Turn off the heat and leave the pan covered so the rice can steam while you cook the squid.

4 Remove the tentacles from the squid and reserve.

5 Cut the body cavity in half. Using the tip of a small, sharp knife, score the inside flesh of the body cavity in a diamond pattern. Do not cut all the way through.

6 Mix the lemon rind, crushed garlic and chopped shallot together.

7 Place all the squid, including the tentacles, in a shallow bowl and sprinkle over the lemon mixture and stir.

8 Heat a griddle pan until almost smoking. Cook the squid for 3–4 minutes until cooked through, then slice.

9 Sprinkle with the coriander and lemon juice. Season to taste with pepper. Drain the rice and serve immediately with the squid.

✓ cows' milk-free　✓ egg-free　✓ gluten-free　✓ wheat-free　✓ nut-free　✓ vegetarian　✓ vegan　✓ seafood-free

Haddock with an Olive Crust

Nutritional details

per 100 g

energy	93 kcals/394 kj
protein	13 g
carbohydrate	6 g
fat	2 g
fibre	1.2 g
sugar	1.1 g
sodium	0.2 g

Ingredients   Serves 4

12 pitted black olives,
  finely chopped
75 g/3 oz fresh white
  breadcrumbs
1 tbsp freshly
  chopped tarragon
1 garlic clove, peeled
  and crushed
3 spring onions, trimmed
  and finely chopped
1 tbsp olive oil
4 x 175 g/6 oz thick skinless
  haddock fillets

To serve:
freshly cooked carrots
freshly cooked beans

Step-by-step guide

1 Preheat the oven to 190°C/
   375°F/Gas Mark 5. Place the black
   olives in a small bowl with the
   breadcrumbs and add the
   chopped tarragon.

2 Add the garlic to the olives with
   the chopped spring onions and
   the olive oil. Mix together lightly.

3 Wipe the fillets with either
   a clean damp cloth or damp
   kitchen paper, then place on a
   lightly oiled baking sheet.

4 Place spoonfuls of the olive and
   breadcrumb mixture on top of
   each fillet and press the mixture
   down lightly and evenly over the
   top of the fish.

5 Bake the fish in the preheated
   oven for 20–25 minutes or until
   the fish is cooked thoroughly and
   the topping is golden brown.
   Serve immediately with the freshly
   cooked carrots and beans.

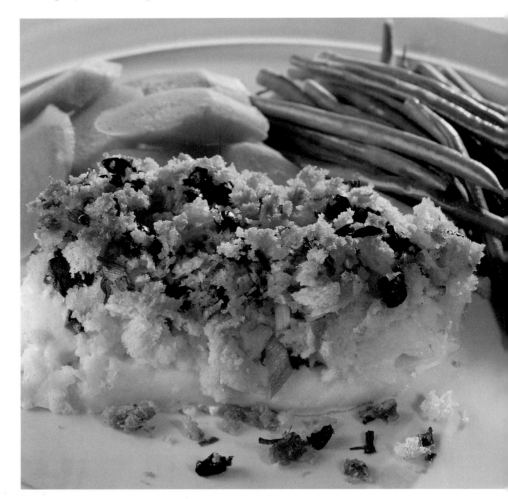

cows' milk-free   egg-free   gluten-free   wheat-free   nut-free   vegetarian   vegan   seafood-free

Hot Salsa-filled Sole

Nutritional details

per 100 g

energy	73 kcals/305 kj
protein	12 g
carbohydrate	4 g
fat	1 g
fibre	trace
sugar	0.3 g
sodium	trace

Ingredients — Serves 4

8 x 175 g/6 oz lemon sole
   fillets, skinned
150 ml/¼ pint orange juice
2 tbsp lemon juice

For the salsa:
1 small, ripe mango
8 cherry tomatoes, quartered
1 small red onion, peeled
   and finely chopped
pinch of sugar
1 red chilli
2 tbsp rice vinegar
zest and juice of 1 lime
1 tbsp olive oil
freshly ground
   black pepper
2 tbsp freshly chopped mint
lime wedges, to garnish
salad leaves, to serve

Step-by-step guide

1 First make the salsa. Peel the mango and cut the flesh away from the stone. Chop finely and place in a small bowl. Add the cherry tomatoes to the mango together with the onion and sugar.

2 Cut the top of the chilli. Slit down the side and discard the seeds and the membrane (the skin to which the seeds are attached). Finely chop the chilli and add to the mango mixture with the vinegar, lime zest, juice and oil. Season to taste with salt and pepper. Mix thoroughly and leave to stand for 30 minutes to allow the flavours to develop.

3 Lay the fish fillets on a board skinned-side up and pile the salsa on the tail end of the fillets. Fold the fillets in half, season and place in a large, shallow frying pan. Pour over the orange and lemon juice.

4 Bring to a gentle boil, then reduce the heat to a simmer. Cover and cook on a low heat for 7–10 minutes, adding a little water if the liquid is evaporating. Remove the cover, add the mint and cook uncovered for a further 3 minutes. Garnish with lime wedges and serve immediately with the salad.

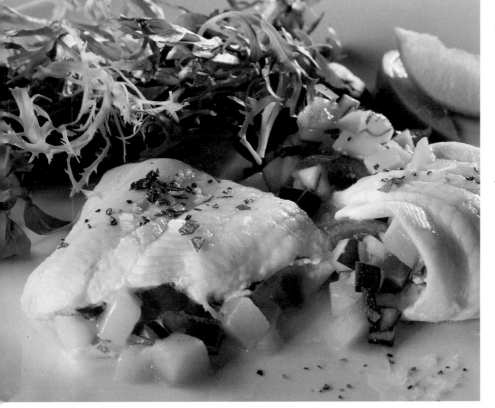

cows' milk-free   egg-free   gluten-free   wheat-free   nut-free   vegetarian   vegan   seafood-free

Jamaican Jerk Pork with Rice & Peas

Nutritional details

per 100 g

energy	117 kcals/492 kj
protein	9 g
carbohydrate	11 g
fat	4 g
fibre	1.2 g
sugar	2.6 g
sodium	0.3 g

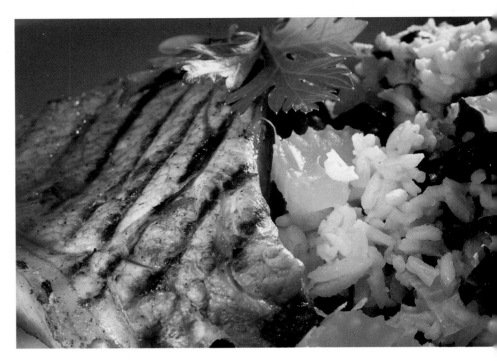

Ingredients   Serves 4

175 g/6 oz dried red kidney beans,
   soaked overnight
2 onions, peeled and chopped
2 garlic cloves, peeled and crushed
4 tbsp lime juice
2 tbsp each dark molasses,
   soy sauce and chopped
   fresh root ginger
2 jalapeño chillies, deseeded
   and chopped
½ tsp ground cinnamon
¼ tsp each ground allspice,
   ground nutmeg
4 pork loin chops, on the bone

For the rice:
1 tbsp vegetable oil
1 onion, peeled and finely chopped
1 celery stalk, trimmed and finely sliced
3 garlic cloves, peeled and crushed
2 bay leaves
225 g/8 oz long-grain white rice
475 ml/18 fl oz chicken or ham stock
sprigs of fresh flat leaf parsley,
   to garnish

Step-by-step guide

1 To make the jerk pork marinade, purée the onions, garlic, lime juice, molasses, soy sauce, ginger, chillies, cinnamon, allspice and nutmeg together in a food processor until smooth. Put the pork chops into a plastic or non-reactive dish and pour over the marinade, turning the chops to coat. Marinate in the refrigerator for at least 1 hour or overnight.

2 Drain the beans and place in a large saucepan with about 2 litres/3½ pints cold water. Bring to the boil and boil rapidly for 10 minutes. Reduce the heat, cover, and simmer gently for 1 hour until tender, adding more water if necessary. When cooked, drain well and mash roughly.

3 Heat the oil for the rice in a saucepan with a tight-fitting lid and add the onion, celery and garlic. Cook gently for 5 minutes until softened. Add the bay leaves, rice and stock and stir. Bring to the boil, cover and cook very gently for 10 minutes. Add the beans and stir well again. Cook for a further 5 minutes, then remove from the heat.

4 Heat a griddle pan until almost smoking. Remove the pork chops from the marinade, scraping off any surplus and add to the hot pan. Cook for 5–8 minutes on each side, or until cooked. Garnish with the parsley and serve immediately with the rice.

Marinated Vegetable Kebabs

Nutritional details

per 100 g

energy	57 kcals/237 kj
protein	2 g
carbohydrate	10 g
fat	1 g
fibre	0.2 g
sugar	0.3 g
sodium	trace

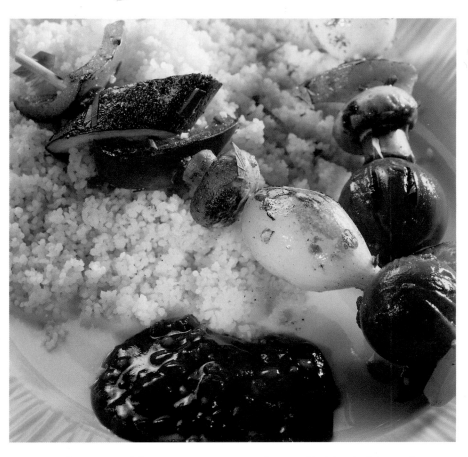

Ingredients   Serves 4

2 small courgettes, cut into
   2 cm/¾ inch pieces
½ green pepper, deseeded and
   cut into 2.5 cm/1 inch pieces
½ red pepper, deseeded and
   cut into 2.5 cm/1 inch pieces
½ yellow pepper, deseeded
   and cut into 2.5 cm/1 inch pieces
8 baby onions, peeled
8 button mushrooms
8 cherry tomatoes
freshly chopped parsley, to garnish
freshly cooked couscous, to serve

For the marinade:
1 tbsp light olive oil
4 tbsp dry sherry
2 tbsp light soy sauce
1 red chilli, deseeded
   and finely chopped
2 garlic cloves, peeled and crushed
2.5 cm/1 inch piece root ginger,
   peeled and finely grated

Step-by-step guide

1 Place the courgettes, peppers and baby onions in a pan of just-boiled water. Bring back to the boil and simmer for about 30 seconds.

2 Drain and rinse the cooked vegetables in cold water and dry on absorbent kitchen paper.

3 Thread the cooked vegetables and the mushrooms and tomatoes alternately on to skewers and place in a large shallow dish.

4 Make the marinade by whisking all the ingredients together until thoroughly blended. Pour the marinade evenly over the kebabs, then chill in the refrigerator for at least 1 hour. Spoon the marinade over the kebabs occasionally during this time.

5 Place the kebabs in a hot griddle pan or on a hot barbecue and cook gently for 10–12 minutes. Turn the kebabs frequently and brush with the marinade when needed. When the vegetables are tender, sprinkle over the chopped parsley and serve immediately with couscous.

✓ cows' milk-free   ✓ egg-free   ✓ gluten-free   ✓ wheat-free   ✓ nut-free   ✓ vegetarian   ✓ vegan   ✓ seafood-free

Mediterranean Potato Salad

Nutritional details

per 100 g

energy	91 kcals/379 kj
protein	2 g
carbohydrate	11 g
fat	5 g
fibre	0.9 g
sugar	2.2 g
sodium	0.2 g

Ingredients   Serves 4

700 g/1½ lb small waxy potatoes
2 red onions, peeled and
    roughly chopped
1 yellow pepper, deseeded
    and roughly chopped
1 green pepper, deseeded and
    roughly chopped
6 tbsp extra-virgin olive oil
125 g/4 oz ripe tomatoes,
    chopped
50 g/2 oz pitted black
    olives, sliced
50 g/2 oz feta cheese
3 tbsp freshly chopped parsley
2 tbsp white wine vinegar
1 tsp Dijon mustard
1 tsp clear honey
freshly ground
    black pepper
sprigs of fresh parsley,
    to garnish

Step-by-step guide

1 Preheat the oven to 200°C/ 400°F/Gas Mark 6. Place the potatoes in a large saucepan of salted water, bring to the boil and simmer until just tender. Do not overcook. Drain and plunge into cold water, to stop them from cooking further.

2 Place the onions in a bowl with the yellow and green peppers, then pour over 2 tablespoons of the olive oil. Stir and spoon onto a large baking tray. Cook in the preheated oven for 25–30 minutes, or until the vegetables are tender and lightly charred in places, stirring occasionally. Remove from the oven and transfer to a large bowl.

3 Cut the potatoes into bite-sized pieces and mix with the roasted onions and peppers. Add the tomatoes and olives to the potatoes. Crumble over the feta cheese and sprinkle with the chopped parsley.

4 Whisk together the remaining olive oil, vinegar, mustard and honey, then season to taste with pepper. Pour the dressing over the potatoes and toss gently together. Garnish with parsley sprigs and serve immediately.

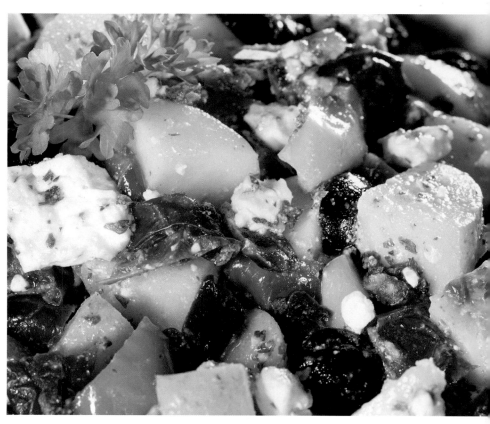

cows' milk-free ✓ egg-free ✓ gluten-free ✓ wheat-free ✓ nut-free ✓ vegetarian ✓ vegan ✓ seafood-free

Mexican Chicken

Nutritional details

per 100 g

energy	139 kcals/586 kj
protein	16 g
carbohydrate	11 g
fat	4 g
fibre	0.4 g
sugar	1.2 g
sodium	0.1 g

      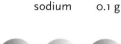

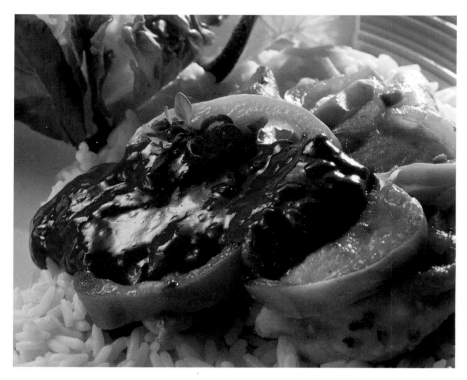

Ingredients — Serves 4

1.4 kg/3 lb oven-ready chicken, jointed
3 tbsp plain flour
½ tsp ground paprika
freshly ground black pepper
2 tsp sunflower oil
1 small onion, peeled and chopped
1 red chilli, deseeded and
   finely chopped
½ tsp ground cumin
½ tsp dried oregano
300 ml/½ pint chicken or
   vegetable stock
1 green pepper, deseeded and sliced
2 tsp cocoa powder
1 tbsp lime juice
2 tsp clear honey
3 tbsp 0%-fat Greek yogurt

To garnish:
sliced limes, red chilli slices
sprig of fresh oregano

To serve:
freshly cooked rice
fresh green salad leaves

Step-by-step guide

1   Using a knife, remove the skin from the chicken joints.

2   In a shallow dish, mix together the flour, paprika and black pepper. Coat the chicken on both sides with flour and shake off any excess if necessary.

3   Heat the oil in a large non-stick frying pan. Add the chicken and brown on both sides. Transfer to a plate and reserve.

4   Add the onion and red chilli to the pan and gently cook for 5 minutes, or until the onion is soft. Stir occasionally.

5   Stir in the cumin and oregano and cook for a further minute. Pour in the stock and bring to the boil.

6   Return the chicken to the pan, cover and cook for 40 minutes. Add the green pepper and cook for 10 minutes, until the chicken is cooked. Remove the chicken and pepper with a slotted spoon and keep warm in a serving dish.

7   Blend the cocoa powder with 1 tablespoon of warm water. Stir into the sauce, then boil rapidly until the sauce has thickened and reduced by about one third. Stir in the lime juice, honey and yogurt.

8   Pour the sauce over the chicken and pepper and garnish with the lime slices, chilli and oregano. Serve immediately with the freshly cooked rice and green salad.

cows' milk-free ✓ egg-free ✓ gluten-free ✓ wheat-free ✓ nut-free ✓ vegetarian ✓ vegan ✓ seafood-free

Mixed Vegetables Stir Fry

Nutritional details

per 100 g

energy	66 kcals/275 kj
protein	2 g
carbohydrate	7 g
fat	4 g
fibre	1.5 g
sugar	4.1 g
sodium	0.3 g

Ingredients   Serves 4

2 tbsp vegetable oil

4 garlic cloves, peeled and
finely sliced

2.5 cm/1 inch piece fresh
root ginger, peeled and
finely sliced

75 g/3 oz broccoli florets

50 g/2 oz mangetout, trimmed

75 g/3 oz carrots, peeled and
cut into matchsticks

1 green pepper, deseeded and
cut into strips

1 red pepper, deseeded and
cut into strips

1 tbsp soy sauce

1 tbsp hoisin sauce

1 tsp sugar

freshly ground
black pepper

4 spring onions,
trimmed and shredded,
to garnish

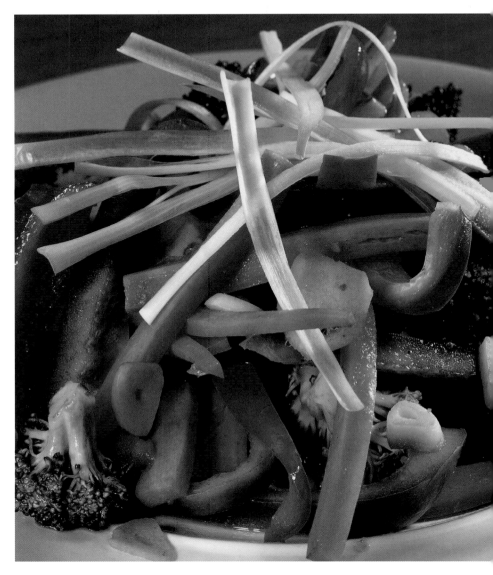

Step-by-step guide

1   Heat a wok, add the oil and when
hot, add the garlic and ginger
slices and stir-fry for 1 minute.

2   Add the broccoli florets to the
wok, stir-fry for 1 minute, then add
the mangetout, carrots and the
green and red peppers and stir-fry
for a further 3–4 minutes, or until
tender but still crisp.

3   Blend the soy sauce, hoisin sauce
and sugar in a small bowl. Stir
well, season to taste with pepper
and pour into the wok. Transfer
the vegetables to a warmed
serving dish. Garnish with
shredded spring onions
and serve immediately.

Pad Thai

Nutritional details

per 100 g

energy	129 kcals/540 kj
protein	13 g
carbohydrate	8 g
fat	5 g
fibre	0.5 g
sugar	2.3 g
sodium	0.6 g

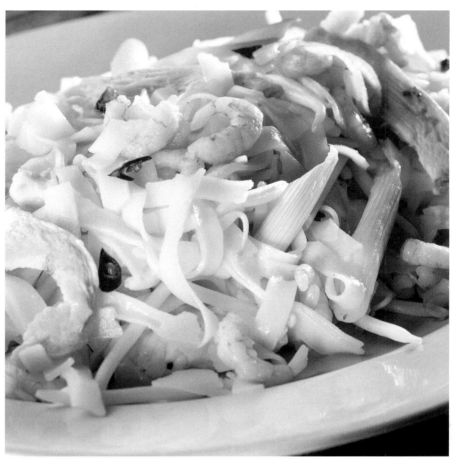

Ingredients   Serves 4

225 g/8 oz flat rice noodles
2 tbsp vegetable oil
225 g/8 oz boneless chicken breast, skinned and thinly sliced
4 shallots, peeled and thinly sliced
2 garlic cloves, peeled and finely chopped
4 spring onions, trimmed and diagonally cut into 5 cm/2 inch pieces
350 g/12 oz fresh white crab meat or tiny prawns
75 g/3 oz fresh bean sprouts, rinsed and drained
2 tbsp preserved or fresh radish
2–3 tbsp roasted peanuts, chopped (optional)

For the sauce:
2 tbsp Thai fish sauce (nam pla)
2–3 tbsp rice vinegar or cider vinegar
1 tbsp chilli bean or oyster sauce
1 tbsp toasted sesame oil
1 tbsp light brown sugar
1 red chilli, deseeded and thinly sliced

Step-by-step guide

1 To make the sauce, whisk all the sauce ingredients in a bowl and reserve. Put the rice noodles in a large bowl and pour over enough hot water to cover. Leave to stand for about 15 minutes until softened. Drain and rinse, then drain again.

2 Heat the oil in a wok over a high heat until hot, but not smoking. Add the chicken strips and stir-fry constantly until they begin to colour. Using a slotted spoon, transfer to a plate. Reduce the heat to medium-high.

3 Add the shallots, garlic and spring onions and stir-fry for 1 minute. Stir in the rice noodles, then the reserved sauce and mix well.

4 Add the reserved chicken strips with the crab meat or prawns, bean sprouts and radish and stir well. Cook for about 5 minutes, stirring frequently, until heated through. If the noodles begin to stick, add a little water.

5 Turn into a large, shallow serving dish and sprinkle with the chopped peanuts, if using. Serve immediately.

cows' milk-free   egg-free   gluten-free   wheat-free   nut-free   vegetarian   vegan   seafood-free

Paella

Nutritional details

per 100 g

energy	92 kcals/384 kj
protein	9 g
carbohydrate	7 g
fat	3 g
fibre	0.7 g
sugar	1.4 g
sodium	0.3 g

Ingredients   Serves 6

450 g/1 lb live mussels
4 tbsp olive oil
6 medium chicken thighs, skinned
1 medium onion, peeled
    and finely chopped
1 garlic clove, peeled and crushed
225 g/8 oz tomatoes, skinned,
    deseeded and chopped
1 red pepper, deseeded and chopped
1 green pepper, deseeded
    and chopped
125 g/4 oz frozen peas
1 tsp paprika
450 g/1 lb Arborio rice
½ tsp turmeric
900 ml/1½ pints chicken stock,
    warmed
175 g/6 oz large peeled prawns
freshly ground black pepper
2 limes
1 lemon
1 tbsp freshly chopped basil
whole, cooked, unpeeled prawns,
    to garnish

Step-by-step guide

1   Rinse the mussels under cold running water, scrubbing well to remove any grit and barnacles, then pull off the hairy 'beards'. Tap any open mussels sharply with a knife, and discard if they refuse to close.

2   Heat the oil in a paella pan or large, heavy-based frying pan and cook the chicken thighs for 10–15 minutes until golden. Remove and keep warm.

3   Fry the onion and garlic in the remaining oil in the pan for 2–3 minutes, then add the tomatoes, peppers, peas and paprika and cook for a further 3 minutes.

4   Add the rice to the pan and return the chicken with the turmeric and half the stock. Bring to the boil and simmer, gradually adding more stock as it is absorbed. Cook for 20 minutes, or until most of the stock has been absorbed and the rice is almost tender.

5   Put the mussels in a large saucepan with 5 cm/2 inches boiling salted water, cover and steam for 5 minutes. Discard any with shells that have not opened, then stir into the rice with the prawns. Season to taste with pepper. Heat through for 2–3 minutes until piping hot. Squeeze the juice from one of the limes over the paella.

6   Cut the remaining limes and the lemon into wedges and arrange on top of the paella. Sprinkle with the basil, garnish with the prawns and serve.

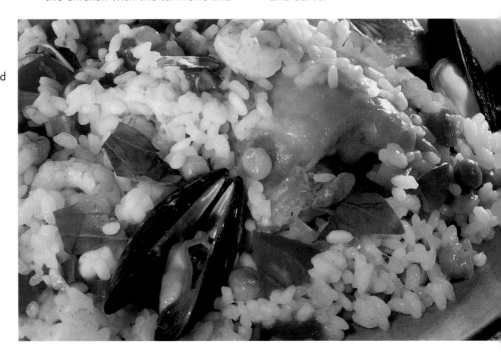

Pasta with Courgettes, Rosemary & Lemon

Nutritional details

per 100 g

energy	85 kcals/360 kj
protein	3 g
carbohydrate	14 g
fat	3 g
fibre	1.1 g
sugar	1 g
sodium	trace

Ingredients   Serves 4

350 g/12 oz dried pasta shapes,
   e.g. rigatoni
1½ tbsp good-quality
   extra virgin olive oil
2 garlic cloves, peeled
   and finely chopped
4 medium courgettes, thinly sliced
1 tbsp freshly chopped rosemary
1 tbsp freshly chopped parsley
zest and juice of 2 lemons
25 g/1 oz pitted black olives,
   roughly chopped
25 g/1 oz pitted green olives,
   roughly chopped
freshly ground black pepper

To garnish:
lemon slices
sprigs of fresh rosemary

Step-by-step guide

1 Bring a large saucepan of salted water to the boil and add the pasta.

2 Return to the boil and cook until 'al dente' or according to the packet instructions.

3 When the pasta is almost done, heat the oil in a large frying pan and add the garlic.

4 Cook over a medium heat until the garlic just begins to brown. Be careful not to overcook the garlic at this stage or it will become bitter.

5 Add the courgettes, rosemary, parsley and lemon zest and juice. Cook for 3–4 minutes until the courgettes are just tender.

6 Add the olives to the frying pan and stir well. Season to taste with pepper and remove from the heat.

7 Drain the pasta well and add to the frying pan. Stir until thoroughly combined. Garnish with lemon and sprigs of fresh rosemary and serve immediately.

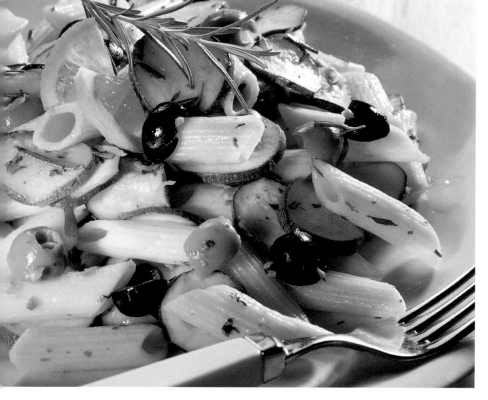

✔ cows' milk-free ✔ egg-free ✔ gluten-free ✔ wheat-free ✔ nut-free ✔ vegetarian ✔ vegan ✔ seafood-free

Peperonata

Nutritional details

per 100 g

energy	52 kcals/217 kj
protein	1 g
carbohydrate	9 g
fat	1 g
fibre	1.3 g
sugar	2.8 g
sodium	trace

Ingredients   Serves 6

2 red peppers
2 yellow peppers
450 g/1 lb waxy potatoes
1 large onion
2 tbsp good quality virgin olive oil
700 g/1½ lb tomatoes, peeled,
    deseeded and chopped
2 small courgettes
50 g/2 oz pitted black
    olives, quartered
small handful basil leaves
freshly ground
    black pepper
crusty bread, to serve

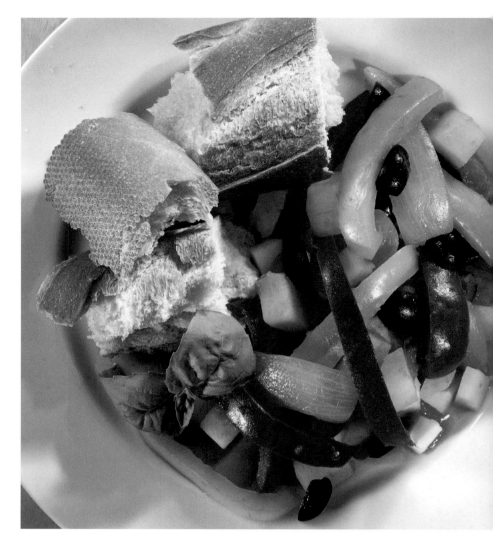

Step-by-step guide

1   Prepare the peppers by halving them lengthwise and removing the stems, seeds, and membranes.

2   Cut the peppers lengthwise into strips about 1 cm/½ inch wide.

Peel the potatoes and cut into rough cubes, about 2.5–3cm/1–1¼ inch across. Cut the onion lengthwise into eight wedges.

3   Heat the olive oil in a large saucepan over a medium heat.

4   Add the onion and cook for about 5 minutes, or until starting to brown.

5   Add the peppers, potatoes, tomatoes, courgettes, black olives and about four torn basil leaves. Season to taste with pepper.

6   Stir the mixture, cover and cook over a very low heat for about 40 minutes, or until the vegetables are tender but still hold their shape. Garnish with the remaining basil. Transfer to a serving bowl and serve immediately, with chunks of crusty bread.

cows' milk-free   egg-free   gluten-free   wheat-free   nut-free   vegetarian   vegan   seafood-free

Pumpkin & Chickpea Curry

Nutritional details

per 100 g

energy	81 kcals/344 kj
protein	3 g
carbohydrate	15 g
fat	2 g
fibre	1.1 g
sugar	1.7 g
sodium	0.1 g

Ingredients   Serves 4

1 tbsp vegetable oil
1 small onion, peeled and sliced
2 garlic cloves, peeled
    and finely chopped
2.5 cm/1 inch piece root ginger,
    peeled and grated
1 tsp ground coriander
½ tsp ground cumin
½ tsp ground turmeric
¼ tsp ground cinnamon
2 tomatoes, chopped
2 red bird's eye chillies,
    deseeded and finely chopped
450 g/1 lb pumpkin
    or butternut squash flesh, cubed
1 tbsp hot curry paste
300 ml/½ pint vegetable stock
1 large firm banana
400 g can chickpeas,
    drained and rinsed
freshly ground black pepper
1 tbsp freshly chopped coriander
coriander sprigs, to garnish
rice or naan bread, to serve

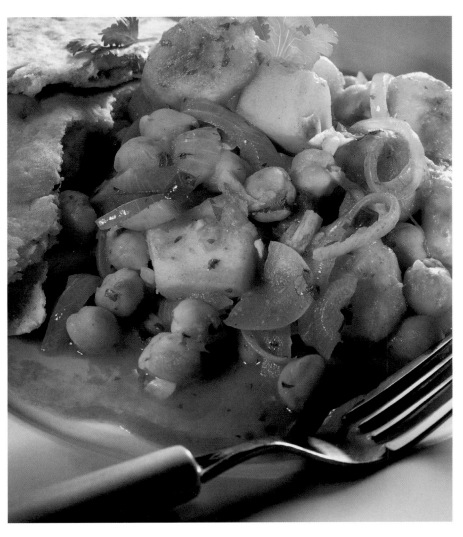

Step-by-step guide

1 Heat 1 tablespoon of the oil in a saucepan and add the onion. Fry gently for 5 minutes until softened.

2 Add the garlic, ginger and spices and fry for a further minute. Add the chopped tomatoes and chillies and cook for another minute.

3 Add the pumpkin and curry paste and fry gently for 3–4 minutes before adding the stock.

4 Stir well, bring to the boil and simmer for 20 minutes until the pumpkin is tender.

5 Thickly slice the banana and add to the pumpkin along with the chickpeas. Simmer for a further 5 minutes.

6 Season to taste with pepper and add the chopped coriander. Serve immediately, garnished with coriander sprigs and some rice or naan bread.

✓ cows' milk-free ✓ egg-free ✓ gluten-free ✓ wheat-free ✓ nut-free ✓ vegetarian ✓ vegan ✓ seafood-free

Ratatouille Mackerel

Nutritional details

per 100 g

energy	135 kcals/564 kj
protein	10 g
carbohydrate	5 g
fat	8 g
fibre	0.5 g
sugar	1.5 g
sodium	trace

Ingredients   Serves 4

1 red pepper
1 tbsp olive oil
1 red onion, peeled
1 garlic clove, peeled and
    thinly sliced
2 courgettes, trimmed and
    cut into thick slices
400 g can chopped tomatoes
freshly ground
    black pepper
4 x 275 g/10 oz small
    mackerel, cleaned and
    heads removed
spray of olive oil
lemon juice for drizzling
12 fresh basil leaves
couscous or rice mixed
    with chopped parsley,
    to serve

Step-by-step guide

1 Preheat the oven to 190°C/
   375°F/Gas Mark 5. Cut the top
   off the red pepper, remove the
   seeds and membrane, then cut
   into chunks. Cut the red onion
   into thick wedges.

2 Heat the oil in a large pan and cook
   the onion and garlic for 5 minutes
   or until beginning to soften.

3 Add the pepper chunks and
   courgettes slices and cook for
   a further 5 minutes.

4 Pour in the chopped tomatoes
   with their juice and cook for a
   further 5 minutes. Season to taste
   with salt and pepper and pour
   into an ovenproof dish.

5 Season the fish with pepper
   and arrange on top of the
   vegetables. Spray with a little
   olive oil and lemon juice. Cover
   and cook in the preheated oven
   for 20 minutes.

6 Remove the cover, add the
   basil leaves and return to the
   oven for a further 5 minutes.
   Serve immediately with couscous
   or rice mixed with parsley.

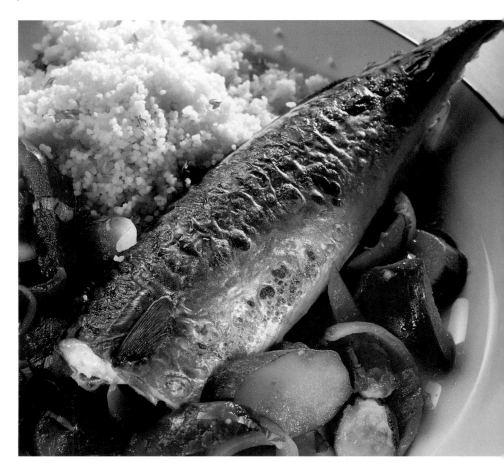

cows' milk-free   egg-free   gluten-free   wheat-free   nut-free   vegetarian   vegan   seafood-free

Rice with Smoked Salmon & Ginger

Nutritional details

per 100 g

energy	123 kcals/517 kj
protein	11 g
carbohydrate	13 g
fat	3 g
fibre	0.2 g
sugar	0.8 g
sodium	1 g

Ingredients   Serves 4

225 g/8 oz basmati rice
600 ml/1 pint fish stock
1 bunch spring onions,
    trimmed and
    diagonally sliced
3 tbsp freshly
    chopped coriander
1 tsp grated fresh
    root ginger
200 g/7 oz sliced
    smoked salmon
1 tbsp soy sauce
1 tsp sesame oil
2 tsp lemon juice
4–6 slices pickled ginger
2 tsp sesame seeds
rocket leaves,
    to serve

Step-by-step guide

1 Place the rice in a sieve and rinse under cold water until the water runs clear. Drain, then place in a large saucepan with the stock and bring gently to the boil. Reduce to a simmer and cover with a tight-fitting lid. Cook for 10 minutes, then remove from the heat and leave, covered, for a further 10 minutes.

2 Stir the spring onions, coriander and fresh ginger into the cooked rice and mix well.

3 Spoon the rice into four tartlet tins, each measuring 10 cm/ 4 inches, and press down firmly with the back of a spoon to form cakes. Invert a tin onto an individual serving plate, then tap the base firmly and remove the tin. Repeat with the rest of the filled tins.

4 Top the rice with the salmon, folding if necessary, so the sides of the rice can still be seen in places. Mix together the soy sauce, sesame oil and lemon juice to make a dressing, then drizzle over the salmon. Top with the pickled ginger and a sprinkling of sesame seeds. Scatter the rocket leaves around the edge of the plates and serve immediately.

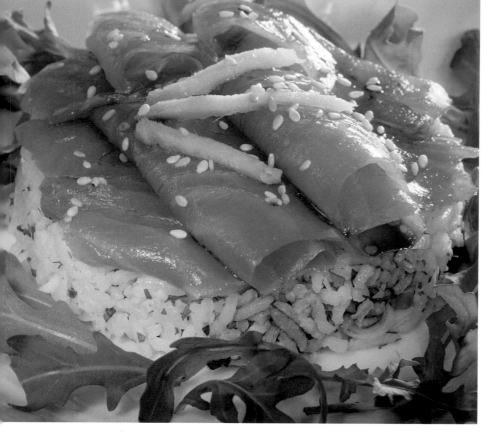

cows' milk-free   egg-free   gluten-free   wheat-free   nut-free   vegetarian   vegan   seafood-free

Rice with Squash & Sage

Nutritional details

per 100 g

energy	107 kcals/446 kj
protein	2 g
carbohydrate	14 g
fat	5 g
fibre	0.2 g
sugar	0.6 g
sodium	0.3 g

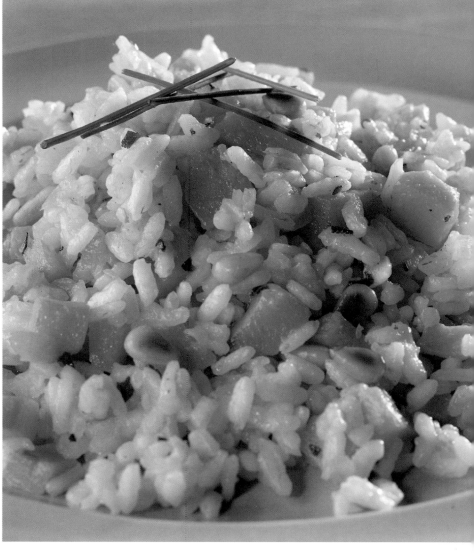

Ingredients   Serves 4–6

450 g/1 lb butternut squash
2 tbsp olive oil
1 small onion, peeled and
    finely chopped
3 garlic cloves, peeled
    and crushed
2 tbsp freshly
    chopped sage
1 litre/1¾ pints vegetable
    stock
450 g/1 lb Arborio rice
50 g/2 oz pine nuts, toasted
freshly snipped chives,
    to garnish
freshly ground
    black pepper

Step-by-step guide

1 Peel the squash, cut in half
   lengthways and remove seeds and
   stringy flesh. Cut remaining flesh
   into small cubes and reserve.

2 Heat the wok, add the oil and heat
   until bubbling, then add the
   onion, garlic and sage and stir-fry
   for 1 minute.

3 Add the squash to the wok and
   stir-fry for a further 10–12
   minutes, or until the squash is
   tender. Remove from the heat.

4 Meanwhile, bring the vegetable or
   chicken stock to the boil and add

the rice. Cook for 8–10 minutes,
or until the rice is just tender but
still quite wet.

5 Add the cooked rice to the squash
   mixture. Stir in the pine nuts and
   season to taste with pepper.
   Garnish with snipped chives and
   serve immediately.

cows' milk-free egg-free gluten-free wheat-free nut-free vegetarian vegan seafood-free

Rich Tomato Soup with Roasted Red Peppers

Nutritional details

per 100 g

energy	42 kcals/175 kj
protein	1 g
carbohydrate	6 g
fat	2 g
fibre	1.5 g
sugar	5.3 g
sodium	0.1 g

Ingredients   Serves 4

2 tsp light olive oil
700 g/1½ lb red peppers,
    halved and deseeded
450 g/1 lb ripe plum
    tomatoes, halved
2 onions, unpeeled and quartered
4 garlic cloves, unpeeled
600 ml/1 pint vegetable stock
salt and freshly ground
    black pepper
4 tbsp soured cream
1 tbsp freshly shredded basil

Step-by-step guide

1   Preheat oven to 200°C/400°F/
Gas Mark 6. Lightly oil a roasting
tin with 1 teaspoon of the olive oil.
Place the peppers and tomatoes

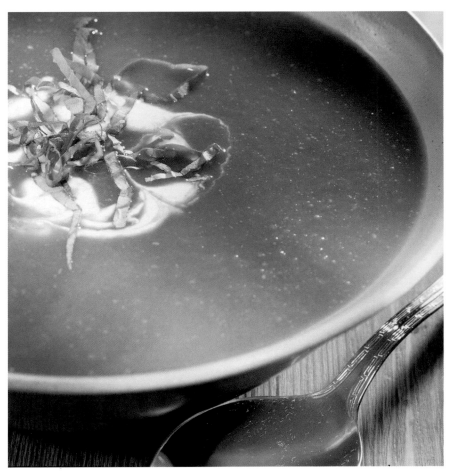

cut-side down in the roasting tin
with the onion quarters and the
garlic cloves. Spoon over the
remaining oil.

2   Bake in the preheated oven for 30
minutes, or until the skins on the
peppers have started to blacken
and blister. Allow the vegetables
to cool for about 10 minutes, then
remove the skins, stalks and
seeds from the peppers. Peel away
the skins from the tomatoes and
onions and squeeze out the garlic.

3   Place the cooked vegetables into a
blender or food processor and
blend until smooth. Add the stock
and blend again to form a smooth
purée. Pour the puréed soup
through a sieve, if a smooth soup
is preferred, then pour into a
saucepan. Bring to the boil,
simmer gently for 2–3 minutes,
and season to taste with salt and
pepper. Serve hot with a swirl of
soured cream and a sprinkling of
shredded basil on the top.

✓ cows' milk-free ✓ egg-free ✓ gluten-free ✓ wheat-free ✓ nut-free ✓ vegetarian ✓ vegan ✓ seafood-free

Salmon Noisettes with Fruity Sauce

Nutritional details

per 100 g

energy	129 kcals/537 kj
protein	10 g
carbohydrate	5 g
fat	9 g
fibre	0.3 g
sugar	2 g
sodium	trace

Ingredients   Serves 4

4 x 125 g/4 oz salmon steaks
grated rind and juice of
    2 lemons
grated rind and juice of
    1 lime
3 tbsp olive oil
1 tbsp clear honey
1 tbsp wholegrain mustard
freshly ground black pepper
1 tbsp sunflower oil
125 g/4 oz mixed salad
    leaves, washed
1 bunch watercress,
    washed and thick
    stalks removed
250 g/9 oz baby plum
    tomatoes, halved

Step-by-step guide

1 Using a sharp knife, cut the bone away from each salmon steak to create two salmon fillets. Repeat with the remaining salmon steaks. Shape the salmon fillets into noisettes and secure with fine string.

2 Mix together the citrus rinds and juices, olive oil, honey, wholegrain mustard and pepper in a shallow dish. Add the salmon fillets and turn to coat. Cover and leave to marinate in the refrigerator for 4 hours, turning them occasionally in the marinade.

3 Heat the wok then add the sunflower oil and heat until hot. Lift out the salmon noisettes, reserving the marinade. Add the salmon to the wok and cook for 6–10 minutes, turning once during cooking, until the fish is cooked through and just flaking. Pour the marinade into the wok and heat through gently.

4 Mix together the salad leaves, watercress and tomatoes and arrange on serving plates. Top with the salmon noisettes and drizzle over any remaining warm marinade. Serve immediately.

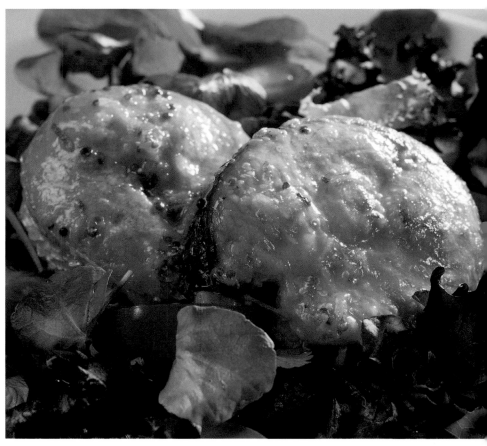

Salmon with Herbed Potatoes

Nutritional details

per 100 g

energy	111 kcals/464 kj
protein	10 g
carbohydrate	6 g
fat	6 g
fibre	1.1 g
sugar	0.9 g
sodium	trace

Ingredients   Serves 4

450 g/1 lb baby
    new potatoes
freshly ground
    black pepper
4 salmon steaks, each weighing
    about 175 g/6 oz
1 carrot, peeled and cut
    into fine strips
175 g/6 oz asparagus
    spears, trimmed
175 g/6 oz sugar snap
    peas, trimmed
finely grated rind and
    juice 1 lemon
1 tbsp olive oil
4 large sprigs of fresh parsley

Step-by-step guide

1   Preheat the oven to 190°C/375°F/ Gas Mark 5, about 10 minutes before required. Parboil the potatoes in lightly salted boiling water for 5–8 minutes until they are barely tender. Drain and reserve.

2   Cut out four pieces of baking parchment paper, measuring 20.5 cm/8 inches square, and place on the work surface. Arrange the parboiled potatoes on top. Wipe the salmon steaks and place on top of the potatoes.

3   Place the carrot strips in a bowl with the asparagus spears, sugar snaps and grated lemon rind and juice. Season to taste with salt and pepper. Toss lightly together.

4   Divide the vegetables evenly between the salmon parcels. Drizzle the top of each parcel with olive oil and add a sprig of parsley.

5   To wrap a parcel, lift up two opposite sides of the paper and fold the edges together. Twist the paper at the other two ends to seal the parcel well. Repeat with the remaining parcels.

6   Place the parcels on a baking tray and bake in the preheated oven for 15 minutes. Place an unopened parcel on each plate and open just before eating.

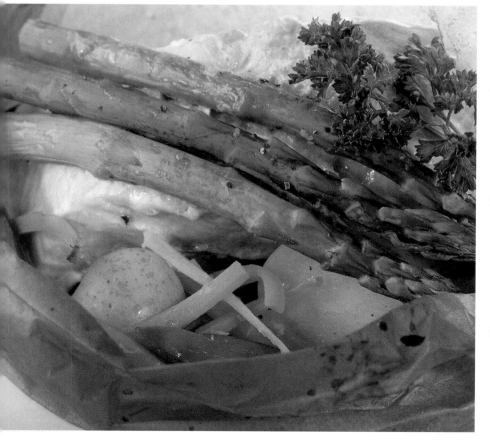

✓ cows' milk-free ✓ egg-free ✓ gluten-free ✓ wheat-free ✓ nut-free ✓ vegetarian ✓ vegan ✓ seafood-free

Sardines with Redcurrants

Nutritional details

per 100 g

energy	137 kcals/573 kj
protein	13 g
carbohydrate	7 g
fat	7 g
fibre	0.2 g
sugar	5 g
sodium	0.1 g

Ingredients   Serves 4

2 tbsp redcurrant jelly
finely grated rind of 1 lime
2 tbsp medium dry sherry
450 g/1 lb fresh sardines,
    cleaned and heads removed
freshly ground
    black pepper
lime wedges, to garnish

To serve:
fresh redcurrants
fresh green salad

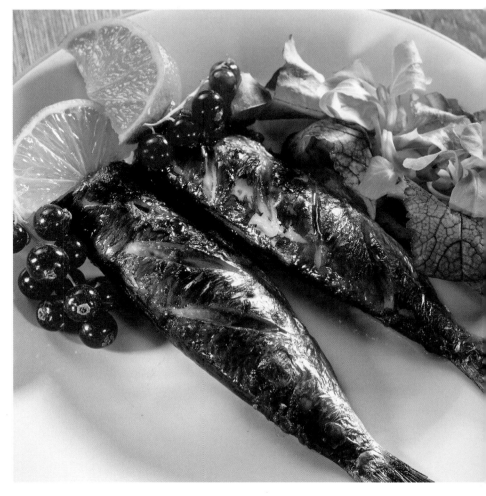

Step-by-step guide

1 Preheat the grill and line the grill rack with tinfoil 2–3 minutes before cooking.

2 Warm the redcurrant jelly in a bowl standing over a pan of gently simmering water and stir until smooth. Add the lime rind and sherry to the bowl and stir well until blended.

3 Lightly rinse the sardines and pat dry with absorbent kitchen paper.

4 Place on a chopping board and with a sharp knife make several diagonal cuts across the flesh of each fish. Season the sardines inside the cavities with pepper.

5 Gently brush the warm marinade over the skin and inside the cavities of the sardines.

6 Place on the grill rack and cook under the preheated grill for 8–10 minutes, or until the fish are cooked.

7 Carefully turn the sardines over at least once during grilling. Baste occasionally with the remaining redcurrant and lime marinade. Garnish with the redcurrants and serve immediately with the salad and lime wedges.

Spiced Couscous & Vegetables

Nutritional details

per 100 g

energy	65 kcals/275 kj
protein	2 g
carbohydrate	12 g
fat	2 g
fibre	0.5 g
sugar	4.3 g
sodium	0.1 g

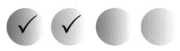

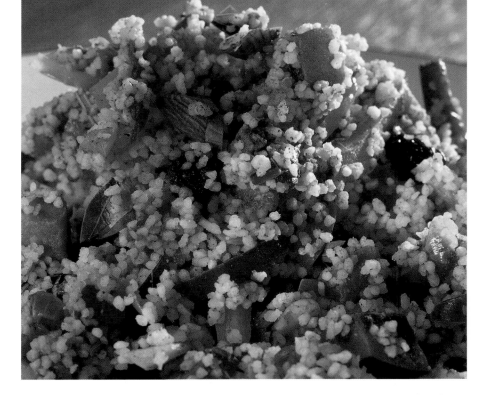

Ingredients Serves 4

1 tbsp olive oil
1 large shallot, peeled
   and finely chopped
1 garlic clove, peeled
   and finely chopped
1 small red pepper, deseeded
   and cut into strips
1 small yellow pepper, deseeded
   and cut into strips
1 small aubergine, diced
1 tsp each turmeric, ground cumin,
   ground cinnamon and paprika
2 tsp ground coriander
large pinch saffron strands
2 tomatoes, peeled,
   deseeded and diced
2 tbsp lemon juice
225 g/8 oz couscous
225 ml/8 fl oz vegetable stock
2 tbsp raisins
2 tbsp whole almonds
2 tbsp freshly chopped parsley
2 tbsp freshly chopped coriander
freshly ground black pepper

Step-by-step guide

1 Heat the oil in a large frying pan
   and add the shallot and garlic and
   cook for 2–3 minutes until
   softened. Add the peppers and
   aubergine and reduce the heat.

2 Cook for 8–10 minutes until the
   vegetables are tender, adding a
   little water if necessary.

3 Test a piece of aubergine to
   ensure it is cooked through.
   Add all the spices and cook for
   a further minute, stirring.

4 Increase the heat and add the
   tomatoes and lemon juice.
   Cook for 2–3 minutes until the
   tomatoes have started to break
   down. Remove from the heat and
   leave to cool slightly.

5 Meanwhile, put the couscous into
   a large bowl. Bring the stock to
   the boil in a saucepan, then pour
   over the couscous. Stir well and
   cover with a clean tea towel.

6 Leave to stand for 7–8 minutes
   until all the stock is absorbed and
   the couscous is tender.

7 Uncover the couscous and fluff
   with a fork. Stir in the vegetable
   and spice mixture along with the
   raisins, almonds, parsley and
   coriander. Season to taste with
   pepper and serve.

Spicy Cucumber Stir Fry

Nutritional details

per 100 g

energy	61 kcals/251 kj
protein	2 g
carbohydrate	3 g
fat	5 g
fibre	0.6 g
sugar	0.2 g
sodium	0.2 g

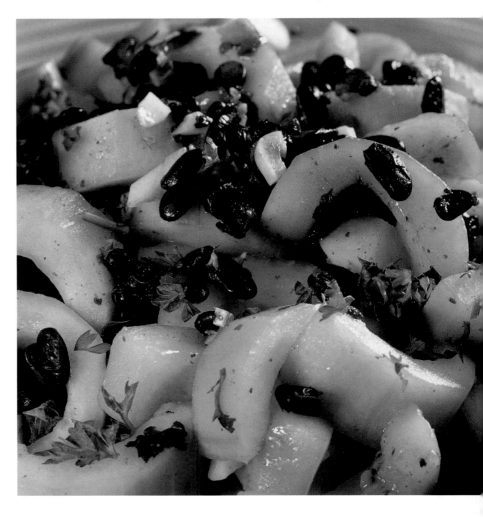

Ingredients Serves 4

25 g/1 oz black soya
    beans, soaked in cold
    water, overnight
1½ cucumbers
1 tbsp vegetable oil
½ tsp mild chilli powder
4 garlic cloves,
    peeled and crushed
5 tbsp vegetable stock
1 tsp sesame oil
1 tbsp freshly chopped
    parsley, to garnish

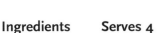

Step-by-step guide

1 Rinse the soaked beans thoroughly,
then drain. Place in a saucepan,
cover with cold water and bring to
the boil, skimming off any scum
that rises to the surface. Boil for
10 minutes, then reduce the heat
and simmer for 1–1½ hours. Drain
and reserve.

2 Peel the cucumbers, slice
lengthways and remove the seeds.
Cut into 2.5 cm/1 inch slices.

3 Heat a wok or large frying pan,
add the oil and when hot, add the
chilli powder, garlic and black
beans and stir-fry for 30 seconds.

4 Add the cucumber and stir-fry
for 20 seconds.

5 Pour the stock into the wok and
cook for 3–4 minutes, or until the
cucumber is very tender. The liquid
will have evaporated at this stage.

6 Remove from the heat and stir in
the sesame oil. Turn into a warmed
serving dish, garnish with chopped
parsley and serve immediately.

Steamed Whole Trout with Ginger & Spring Onion

Nutritional details

per 100 g

energy	147 kcals/619 kj
protein	15 g
carbohydrate	9 g
fat	6 g
fibre	trace
sugar	trace
sodium	trace

Ingredients　　Serves 4

2 x 450–700 g/1–1½ lb whole trout,
　gutted with heads removed
2 tbsp sunflower oil
½ tbsp soy sauce
1 tbsp sesame oil
2 garlic cloves, peeled and
　thinly sliced
2.5 cm/1 inch piece fresh root ginger,
　peeled and thinly slivered
2 spring onions, trimmed
　and thinly sliced diagonally

To garnish:
chive leaves
lemon slices

To serve:
freshly cooked rice
Oriental salad, to serve

Step-by-step guide

1　Wipe the fish inside and out with absorbent kitchen paper.

2　Set a steamer rack or inverted ramekin in a large wok and pour in enough water to come about 5 cm/2 inches up the side of the wok. Bring to the boil.

3　Brush a heatproof dinner plate with a little of the sunflower oil and place the fish on the plate with the tails pointing in opposite directions. Place the plate on the rack, cover tightly and simmer over a medium heat for 10–12 minutes, or until tender and the flesh is opaque near the bone.

4　Carefully transfer the plate to a heatproof surface. Sprinkle with the soy sauce and keep warm.

5　Pour the water out of the wok and return to the heat. Add the remaining sunflower and sesame oils and when hot, add the garlic, ginger and spring onion and stir-fry for 2 minutes, or until golden. Pour over the fish, garnish with chive leaves and lemon slices and serve immediately with rice and an Oriental salad.

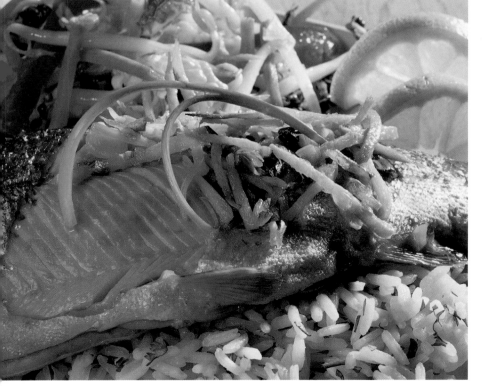

✓ cows' milk-free　✓ egg-free　✓ gluten-free　✓ wheat-free　✓ nut-free　✓ vegetarian　✓ vegan　✓ seafood-free

Stir-fried Chicken with Spinach, Tomatoes & Pine Nuts

Nutritional details

per 100 g

energy	120 kcals/503 kj
protein	10 g
carbohydrate	9 g
fat	5 g
fibre	1.2 g
sugar	3.7 g
sodium	trace

Ingredients   Serves 4

50 g/2 oz pine nuts
2 tbsp sunflower oil
1 red onion, peeled and
    finely chopped
450 g/1 lb skinless, boneless
    chicken breast fillets,
    cut into strips
450 g/1 lb cherry
    tomatoes, halved
225 g/8 oz baby
    spinach, washed
freshly ground
    black pepper
¼ tsp freshly grated nutmeg
2 tbsp balsamic vinegar
50 g/2 oz raisins
freshly cooked ribbon noodles,
    to serve

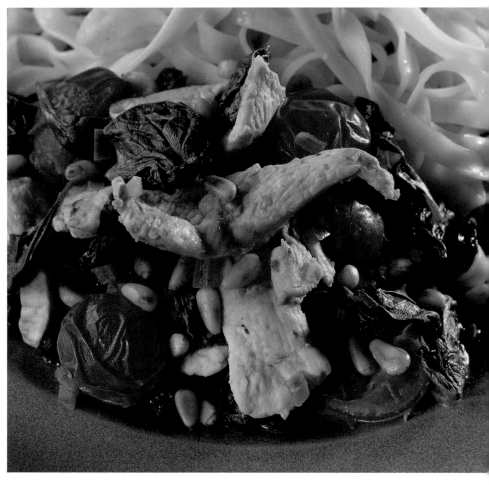

Step-by-step guide

1. Heat the wok and add the pine nuts. Dry-fry for about 2 minutes, shaking often to ensure that they toast but do not burn. Remove and reserve. Wipe any dust from the wok.

2. Heat the wok again, add the oil and when hot, add the red onion and stir-fry for 2 minutes. Add the chicken and stir-fry for 2–3 minutes, or until golden brown.

Reduce the heat, toss in the cherry tomatoes and stir-fry gently until the tomatoes start to disintegrate.

3. Add the baby spinach and stir-fry for 2–3 minutes, or until they start to wilt. Season to taste with pepper, then sprinkle in the grated nutmeg and drizzle in the balsamic vinegar. Finally, stir in the raisins and reserved toasted pine nuts. Serve immediately on a bed of ribbon noodles.

cows' milk-free   egg-free   gluten-free   wheat-free   nut-free   vegetarian   vegan   seafood-free

Thai Noodles & Vegetables with Tofu

Nutritional details

per 100 g

energy	52 kcals/218 kj
protein	4 g
carbohydrate	7 g
fat	1 g
fibre	0.4 g
sugar	0.5 g
sodium	0.3 g

Ingredients   Serves 4

225 g/8 oz firm tofu
1 tbsp soy sauce
rind of 1 lime, grated
2 lemon grass stalks
1 red chilli
1 litre/1¾ pint vegetable stock
2 slices fresh root
    ginger, peeled
2 garlic cloves, peeled
2 sprigs of fresh coriander
175 g/6 oz dried thread
    egg noodles
125 g/4 oz shiitake or button
    mushrooms, sliced if large
2 carrots, peeled and
    cut into matchsticks
125 g/4 oz mangetout
125 g/4 oz pak choi or
    other Chinese leaf
1 tbsp freshly chopped coriander
freshly ground
    black pepper
coriander sprigs, to garnish

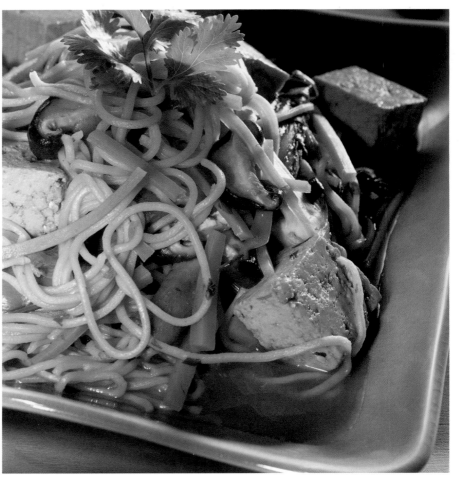

Step-by-step guide

1   Drain the tofu well and cut into cubes. Put into a shallow dish with the soy sauce and lime rind. Stir well to coat and leave to marinate for 30 minutes.

2   Meanwhile, put the lemon grass and chilli on a chopping board and bruise with the side of a large knife, ensuring the blade is pointing away from you. Put the vegetable stock in a large saucepan and add the lemon grass, chilli, ginger, garlic, and coriander. Bring to the boil, cover and simmer gently for 20 minutes.

3   Strain the stock into a clean pan. Return to the boil and add the noodles, tofu and its marinade and the mushrooms. Simmer gently for 4 minutes.

4   Add the carrots, mangetout, pak choi and coriander and simmer for a further 3–4 minutes until the vegetables are just tender. Season to taste with pepper, garnish with coriander sprigs and serve immediately.

cows' milk-free   egg-free   gluten-free   wheat-free   nut-free   vegetarian   vegan   seafood-free

Thai Stir-fried Noodles

Nutritional details

per 100 g

energy	141 kcals/588 kj
protein	11 g
carbohydrate	5 g
fat	9 g
fibre	0.8 g
sugar	2.1 g
sodium	0.1 g

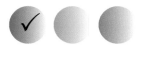

Step-by-step guide

1 Cut the tofu into cubes and place in a bowl. Sprinkle over the sherry and toss to coat. Cover loosely and leave to marinate in the refrigerator for 30 minutes.

2 Bring a large saucepan of lightly salted water to the boil and add the noodles and mangetout. Simmer for 3 minutes or according to the packet instructions, then drain and rinse under cold running water. Leave to drain again.

3 Heat a wok or large frying pan, add the oil and when hot, add the onion and stir-fry for 2–3 minutes. Add the garlic and ginger and stir-fry for 30 seconds. Add the beansprouts and tofu, stir in the Thai fish sauce and the soy sauce with the sugar and season to taste with pepper.

4 Stir-fry the tofu mixture over a medium heat for 2–3 minutes, then add the courgettes, noodles and mangetout and stir-fry for a further 1–2 minutes. Tip into a warmed serving dish or spoon on to individual plates. Sprinkle with the peanuts, add a sprig of basil and serve immediately.

Ingredients   Serves 4

450 g/1 lb tofu
2 tbsp dry sherry
125 g/4 oz medium egg noodles
125 g/4 oz mangetout, halved
3 tbsp groundnut oil
1 onion, peeled and finely sliced
1 garlic clove, peeled and
    finely sliced
2.5 cm/1 inch piece fresh
    root ginger, peeled and
    finely sliced
125 g/4 oz beansprouts
1 tbsp Thai fish sauce
1 tbsp light soy sauce
½ tsp sugar
freshly ground
    black pepper
½ courgette, cut into matchsticks

To garnish:
2 tbsp roasted peanuts,
    roughly chopped
sprigs of fresh basil

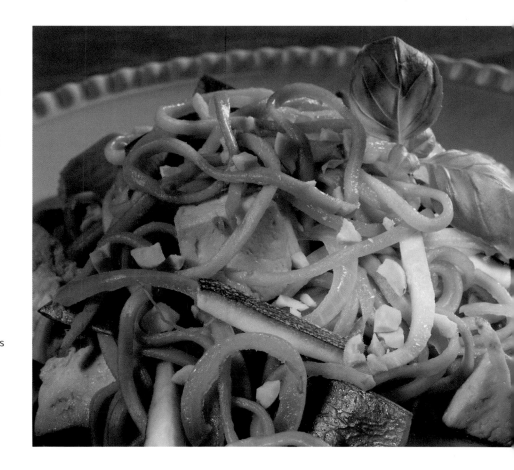

Turkey & Tomato Tagine

Nutritional details

per 100 g

energy	94 kcals/394 kj
protein	12 g
carbohydrate	8 g
fat	2 g
fibre	0.5 g
sugar	1.7 g
sodium	trace

Ingredients   Serves 4

For the meatballs:
450 g/1 lb fresh turkey mince
1 small onion, peeled and
    very finely chopped
1 garlic clove, peeled
    and crushed
1 tbsp freshly chopped coriander
1 tsp ground cumin
1 tbsp olive oil
freshly ground
    black pepper

For the sauce:
1 onion, peeled and finely chopped
1 garlic clove, peeled and crushed
150 ml/¼ pint turkey stock
400 g can chopped tomatoes
½ tsp ground cumin
½ tsp ground cinnamon
pinch of cayenne pepper
freshly chopped parsley
freshly chopped herbs, to garnish
freshly cooked couscous or rice,
    to serve

Step-by-step guide

1   Preheat the oven to 190°C/
    375°F/Gas Mark 5. Put all the
    ingredients for the meatballs
    in a bowl, except the oil and mix
    well. Season to taste with salt
    and pepper. Shape into 20 balls,
    about the size of walnuts.

2   Put on a tray, cover lightly and
    chill in the refrigerator while
    making the sauce.

3   Put the onion and garlic in a pan
    with 125 ml/4 fl oz of the stock.
    Cook over a low heat until all the
    stock has evaporated. Continue
    cooking for 1 minute, or until the
    onions begin to colour.

4   Add the remaining stock to the
    pan with the tomatoes, cumin,
    cinnamon and cayenne pepper.
    Simmer for 10 minutes, until
    slightly thickened and reduced. Stir
    in the parsley and season to taste.

5   Heat the oil in a large, non-stick
    frying pan and cook the meatballs
    in two batches until lightly
    browned all over.

6   Lift the meatballs out with a slotted
    spoon and drain on kitchen paper.

7   Pour the sauce into a tagine or an
    ovenproof casserole. Top with the
    meatballs, cover and cook in the
    preheated oven for 25–30 minutes,
    or until the meatballs are cooked
    through and the sauce is bubbling.
    Garnish with freshly chopped herbs
    and serve immediately on a bed of
    couscous or plain boiled rice.

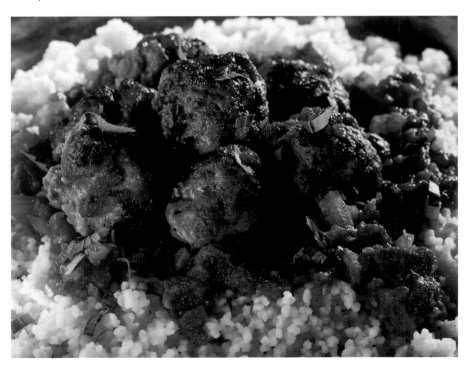

cows' milk-free   egg-free   gluten-free   wheat-free   nut-free   vegetarian   vegan   seafood-free

Turkey with Oriental Mushrooms

Nutritional details

per 100 g

energy	87 kcals/366 kj
protein	10 g
carbohydrate	8 g
fat	2 g
fibre	0.7 g
sugar	1.1 g
sodium	0.1 g

Ingredients   Serves 4

15 g/½ oz dried
     Chinese mushrooms
450 g/1 lb turkey breast steaks
150 ml/¼ pint turkey or
     chicken stock
2 tbsp sunflower oil
1 red pepper, deseeded
     and sliced
225 g/8 oz sugar snap
     peas, trimmed
125 g/4 oz shiitake mushrooms,
     wiped and halved
125 g/4 oz oyster mushrooms,
     wiped and halved
2 tbsp yellow bean sauce
1 tbsp soy sauce
1 tbsp hot chilli sauce
freshly cooked noodles,
     to serve

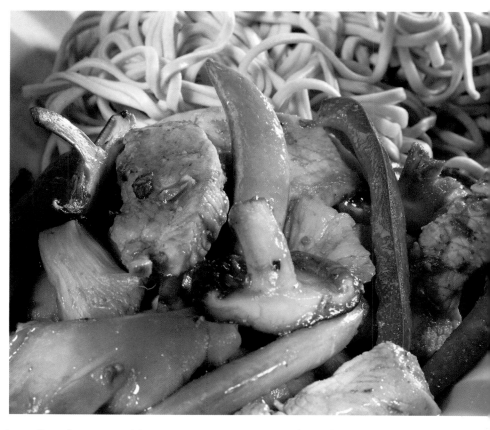

Step-by-step guide

1   Place the dried mushrooms in a small bowl, cover with almost boiling water and leave for 20–30 minutes. Drain and discard any woody stems from the mushrooms. Cut the turkey into thin strips.

2   Pour the turkey or chicken stock into a wok or large frying pan and bring to the boil. Add the turkey and cook gently for 3 minutes, or until the turkey is sealed completely, then using a slotted spoon, remove from the wok and reserve. Discard any stock.

3   Wipe the wok clean and reheat, then add the oil. When the oil is almost smoking, add the drained turkey and stir-fry for 2 minutes.

4   Add the drained mushrooms to the wok with the red pepper, the sugar snap peas and the shiitake and oyster mushrooms. Stir-fry for 2 minutes, then add the yellow bean, soy and hot chilli sauces.

5   Stir-fry the mixture for 1–2 minutes more, or until the turkey is cooked thoroughly and the vegetables are cooked but still retain a bite. Turn into a warmed serving dish and serve immediately with freshly cooked noodles.

cows' milk-free   egg-free   gluten-free   wheat-free   nut-free   vegetarian   vegan   seafood-free

Zesty Whole-baked Fish

Nutritional details

per 100 g

energy	193 kcals/805 kj
protein	21 g
carbohydrate	2 g
fat	12 g
fibre	0.1 g
sugar	0.4 g
sodium	0.2 g

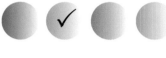
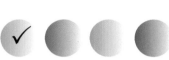

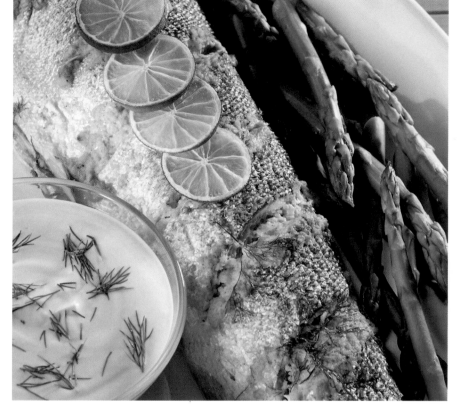

Ingredients   Serves 8

1.8 kg/4 lb whole salmon, cleaned
freshly ground
    black pepper
50 g/2 oz low-fat spread
1 garlic clove, peeled and
    finely sliced
zest and juice of 1 lemon
zest of 1 orange
1 tsp freshly grated nutmeg
3 tbsp Dijon mustard
2 tbsp fresh white breadcrumbs
2 bunches fresh dill
1 bunch fresh tarragon
1 lime sliced
150 ml/¼ pint half-fat crème fraîche
450 ml/¾ pint fromage frais
dill sprigs, to garnish

Step-by-step guide

1   Preheat the oven to 220°C/425°F/
Gas Mark 7. Lightly rinse the fish
and pat dry with absorbent
kitchen paper. Season the cavity
with a little pepper. Make several
diagonal cuts across the flesh of
the fish and season.

2   Mix together the low-fat spread,
garlic, lemon and orange zest and
juice, nutmeg, mustard and fresh
breadcrumbs. Mix well together.
Spoon the breadcrumb mixture
into the slits with a small sprig of
dill. Place the remaining herbs
inside the fish cavity. Weigh the fish
and calculate the cooking time –
allow 10 minutes per 450 g/1 lb.

3   Lay the fish on a double thickness
of tinfoil. If liked, smear the fish
with a little low fat spread. Top
with the lime slices and fold the
foil into a parcel. Chill in the
refrigerator for about 15 minutes.

4   Place in a roasting tin and cook
in the preheated oven for the
calculated cooking time. Fifteen
minutes before the end of
cooking, open the foil and return
until the skin begins to crisp.
Remove the fish from the oven
and stand for 10 minutes.

5   Pour the juices from the roasting
tin into a saucepan. Bring to the
boil and stir in the crème fraîche
and fromage frais. Simmer for 3
minutes or until hot. Garnish with
dill sprigs and serve immediately.

cows' milk-free   egg-free   gluten-free   wheat-free   nut-free   vegetarian   vegan   seafood-free